DRUG IMPORTATION: THE REALITIES OF SAFETY AND SECURITY

WEDNESDAY, FEBRUARY 16, 2005

U.S. SENATE,
COMMITTEE ON HEALTH, EDUCATION, LABOR, AND PENSIONS,
Washington, D.C.

The committee met, pursuant to notice, at 10:01 a.m. in room SD–430, Dirksen Senate Office Building, Hon. Mike Enzi (chairman of the committee) presiding.

Present: Senators Enzi, Alexander, Burr, Kennedy, and Murray.

OPENING STATEMENT OF SENATOR ENZI

The CHAIRMAN. I will go ahead and call to order this hearing on Drug Importation: The Realities of Safety and Security.

Our real purpose in having this series of hearings that we are going to be having is to find out as much as we can about drug reimportation before we do legislation. I know in the ether of Washington, where there are ideas just zipping around in the air all the time, it is kind of hard to hold up and get the information before we grab the answers out of the air, but that is what we are going to try to do with this series, and of course, today, we will focus on the recently released report by a Health and Human Services task force on drug importation that was mandated by the Medicare Modernization Act, and tomorrow, we will be looking at the Department of Commerce's report on price controls overseas and their implications for American consumers.

We want to get into all of the aspects of the drug industry that we possibly can. They have done a marvelous job on coming up with treatments for virtually every disease or on the way to getting one for every disease, both treatment and prevention. I have noticed that there is a relationship between the number of people affected and the price that can be charged and whether there is a solution out there yet for that particular illness.

It all has to be balanced with how we are affected by our need for pharmacists in the United States, and of course, I am a big believer in Main Street and the relationship between the pharmacist and the individual, and I am real pleased with the program that they have where they help review the prescriptions that people have and, in some cases, suggest generics, and at any rate, are saving millions of dollars for people across the United States through that mechanism.

People probably would not even be considering ordering drugs from overseas, except that we have gotten used to using the Internet and have found advantages that the Internet provides, so I do believe that we can develop an import plan to import prescription drugs from other countries and still maintain the level of safety and effectiveness that Americans have come to expect and demand. In fact, drug reimportation probably cannot happen unless we can guarantee those things.

So today, we are taking the first step in this process and focusing our attention on the results of this study. The task force did identify challenges that we have to address if we are to create a feasible drug importation system, and this will give us the opportunity to examine the results of the report in detail.

I appreciate all those who will be testifying today. If we are going to open our borders to prescription medications, we had better be sure how we are going to do it and how it will operate, both in the short-term and in the long run. We have to do it right, and getting our questions answered today will be the first step in that process.

Senator Kennedy.

Opening Statement of Senator Kennedy

Senator KENNEDY. Thank you. Thank you very much, Mr. Chairman.

I want to thank our Chairman Enzi for having this series of hearings. As he has pointed out, drug importation has been an issue that we have considered on the floor. Legislation has been introduced. Unlike many other times when we are considering public policy, we have the examples of what is happening out in the real world in a number of communities, in a number of States around our country.

The United States spend the most in investing in prescription drugs. We then develop these drugs, and I am a great believer that we are living in the period of the life sciences. What we have seen achieved in recent years I think will pale to what the potential breakthroughs will be in these next several years, and the impact on life and on our families, I think, is just going to be extraordinary. If we get a breakthrough with Alzheimer's, we will empty two-thirds of the hospital beds in my State of Massachusetts. The opportunities that are out there are just breathtaking.

But as we spend the most, we also charge the most, and we know that there are similar or the same drugs that are being sold in other countries that are vastly more reasonable and at a lesser price. The real question that our seniors have gotten way ahead of the political leadership on, and understand, is why should we not be able to take advantage of these?

We hear a lot of reasons for it, safety being the most compelling, as well as the impact of taking this course of action on profits and what that will mean in terms of breakthrough on future drugs. We can examine that issue, which we have been unable to really understand completely over the 40 years I have been in the United States Senate, and I doubt if we will ever be able completely to understand that whole issue of profits and the companies.

But we have seen some extraordinary efforts by communities. In Massachusetts, the city of Springfield has been using Canadian pharmacies to provide prescription drugs for its city employees and retirees. Springfield's example led the way for other cities such as

S. HRG. 109–70

DRUG IMPORTATION: THE REALITIES OF SAFETY AND SECURITY

HEARING

BEFORE THE

COMMITTEE ON HEALTH, EDUCATION, LABOR, AND PENSIONS UNITED STATES SENATE

ONE HUNDRED NINTH CONGRESS

FIRST SESSION

ON

EXAMINING THE REALITIES OF SAFETY AND SECURITY REGARDING DRUG IMPORTATION

FEBRUARY 16, 2005

Printed for the use of the Committee on Health, Education, Labor, and Pensions

U.S. GOVERNMENT PRINTING OFFICE

98–923 PDF WASHINGTON : 2005

For sale by the Superintendent of Documents, U.S. Government Printing Office
Internet: bookstore.gpo.gov Phone: toll free (866) 512–1800; DC area (202) 512–1800
Fax: (202) 512–2250 Mail: Stop SSOP, Washington, DC 20402–0001

COMMITTEE ON HEALTH, EDUCATION, LABOR, AND PENSIONS

JUDD GREGG, New Hampshire, *Chairman*

BILL FRIST, Tennessee
MICHAEL B. ENZI, Wyoming
LAMAR ALEXANDER, Tennessee
CHRISTOPHER S. BOND, Missouri
MIKE DeWINE, Ohio
PAT ROBERTS, Kansas
JEFF SESSIONS, Alabama
JOHN ENSIGN, Nevada
LINDSEY GRAHAM, South Carolina
JOHN WARNER, Virginia

EDWARD M. KENNEDY, Massachusetts
CHRISTOPHER J. DODD, Connecticut
TOM HARKIN, Iowa
BARBARA A. MIKULSKI, Maryland
JAMES M. JEFFORDS (I), Vermont
JEFF BINGAMAN, New Mexico
PATTY MURRAY, Washington
JACK REED, Rhode Island
JOHN EDWARDS, North Carolina
HILLARY RODHAM CLINTON, New York

SHARON R. SODERSTROM, *Staff Director*
J. MICHAEL MYERS, *Minority Staff Director and Chief Counsel*

C O N T E N T S

STATEMENTS

WEDNESDAY, FEBRUARY 16, 2005

	Page
Enzi, Hon. Michael B., a U.S. Senator from the State of Wyoming	1
Kennedy, Hon. Edward M., a U.S. Senator from the State of Massachusetts	2
Carmona, Hon. Richard, M.D., M.P.H., F.A.C.S., Surgeon General, U.S. Public Health Service, Department of Health and Human Services, Washington, DC	4
Prepared statement	14
Pawlenty, Hon. Tim, Governor of the State of Minnesota, St. Paul, MN	18
Prepared statement	19
Gray, John M., President and CEO, Healthcare Distribution Management Association (HDMA), Reston, VA	22
Prepared statement	24
Catizone, Carmen A., MS, RPh, DPh, Executive Director/Secretary, National Association of Boards of Pharmacy	27
Prepared statement	29
Rost, Peter, M.D., Vice President of Marketing for Endocrine Care, Pfizer	34
Prepared statement	35

Additional Material

Statements, articles, publications, letters, etc.:	
Pfizer, Inc.	45
Vitter, David, a U.S. Senator from the State of Louisiana, prepared statement	48
American Pharmacists Association (APhA)	49
Allergan, Inc.	52
Response to Questions of Senator Kennedy by Richard Carmona	54
Response to Questions of Senator Hatch by Richard Carmona	55
Response to Questions of Senator Enzi by Carmen Catizone	56
Response to Questions of Senator Enzi by John Gray	56
Response to Questions of Senator Enzi by Governor Tim Pawlenty	57
Response to Questions of Senator Hatch by Governor Tim Pawlenty	59
Response to Questions of the Committee by Peter Rost, M.D.	60

Boston to do the same, and whole States are involved as well, as Governor Pawlenty will tell us. The Internet revolution, as the Chairman mentioned, vastly expanded the opportunity, enabling patients across America to go to Canada on the Internet and save thousands of dollars a year on prescriptions. Meanwhile, the European Union has had parallel trade in drugs, one member nation to another, for decades, and as we will hear from Dr. Rost, parallel trade in Europe is safe, and it saves money.

American experiences such as Springfield's and Minnesota's and the European experience with parallel trade show us that we can import drugs safely and that importation will make drugs more affordable. Access to affordable drugs is critical to patients, in Springfield and in Boston and every city and town in Massachusetts; in fact, it is critical to patients in every American State.

Senators Dorgan, Snowe, Grassley, McCain, Jeffords, Clinton, Bingaman and I introduced last week S. 334 to allow the importation of safe, FDA-approved drugs manufactured in plants inspected by the FDA, and we hope it will be enacted quickly this year. It will allow American patients to buy safe drugs at the fair price that Canadians and Europeans pay, not the exorbitant prices that patients are forced to pay here in the United States.

Finally, President Bush has threatened to veto any attempt to change the new Medicare prescription drug law, and I agree that nothing should be done to weaken an already weak drug benefit. We are talking today about the safe importation of prescription drugs from Canada and Europe, but I believe that the White House should consider an additional common sense step as well to curb the costs of the new Medicare law and ensure a better drug benefit for seniors and the disabled.

By allowing the Medicare program to negotiate fair prices with drug manufacturers, we could save up to $190 billion over the next decades. The Veterans Administration has such negotiating authority and it has used it wisely to cut costs and help our veterans with their prescription drug needs, and I believe that this is a practical step the White House should consider as well.

I want to join in welcoming our Surgeon General Carmona and Governor Pawlenty and our other witnesses today, and I again express appreciation to our Chair for having this hearing. Thank you.

The CHAIRMAN. Well, I thank you, and thank you for the bill that you have submitted and the other bills that have been submitted by other individuals dealing with drug reimportation. I think that from the range of interest that we have on it, we will be able to come up with some good conclusions.

I particularly want to thank Dr. Carmona, the Surgeon General, for his work on the special task force that came up with the drug importation report. I thank him for summarizing it in his testimony and then I hesitate but will ask that he summarize the summarization, assuming that everyone who has been here today will have already read both the full report and your summary so that we can get—I know there are a lot of questions that people have that they are really interested in directing at you, so we appreciate that opportunity.

Dr. Carmona.

STATEMENT OF HON. RICHARD CARMONA, M.D., M.P.H., F.A.C.S., SURGEON GENERAL, U.S. PUBLIC HEALTH SERVICE, DEPARTMENT OF HEALTH AND HUMAN SERVICES, WASHINGTON, DC

Dr. CARMONA. Thank you, Mr. Chairman and Senator Kennedy, other distinguished members of the committee.

Thank you for asking me to join you today. My name is Richard Carmona. I am the United States Surgeon General. I was also the chairman of the HHS Task Force on Drug Importation, which was comprised of 13 senior executives with diverse experience from across the Federal Government. In February 2004, then-Secretary Tommy Thompson created the task force to advise him on questions posed by Congress in the Medicare Modernization Act about the safety issues surrounding the importation of prescription drugs.

As you know, the role of the Surgeon General is to protect and promote the health and well-being of the American people. Everything I do as Surgeon General is based in science, and that was my guiding principle in leading this task force. We went where the facts and the science led us. In doing so, we also ensured an open and transparent process. The task force held six listening sessions, heard from more than 100 presenters, and received information from over 100 individuals and organizations via our online docket.

In addition, I led a site visit to the John F. Kennedy International Airport in New York City to see how imported drugs are processed by U.S. Customs and Border Protection and by officials of the Food and Drug Administration. The visit demonstrated to us the huge challenge of ensuring the safety of imported drugs.

After that site visit and after listening to all of the presenters, reading the statements and studying the science, the task force produced a comprehensive 127-page report. The report has eight key findings. They are: our current system of drug regulation has been very effective in protecting the public safety, but it is facing new threats. Any change to our current regulatory system must be done with great care to ensure the continued safety and efficacy of our Nation's drug supply.

Two, there are significant risks associated with the current illegal importation of drugs for personal use. To name just a few, there are 355 points of entry for access into the United States. This includes 14 international mail branches, 29 express consignment facilities and 312 ports. FDA inspectors are already stretched thin reviewing the millions of prescription drug packages that currently pass through those points of entry each year.

We all know that illegally purchasing prescription drugs over the Internet without a prescription is relatively easy to do. The reality is that this lack of relationship between a doctor and a patient is extremely dangerous and potentially fatal. Although some licensed Internet pharmacies provide a legitimate way to buy medicines, many Internet pharmacies are not licensed. They are rogue operations that pretend to be legitimate and are actually providing dangerous products, and by dangerous, I mean that these drugs are often grossly mislabeled, expired, subpotent, superpotent or placebos and have usually been transported improperly with a complete disregard for safety precautions.

Three, the task force found that it would be extraordinarily difficult and costly for personal importation to be implemented in a way that would ensure the safety and effectiveness of all prescription drugs.

Four, looking at commercial prescription drug importation, the overall national savings would likely be small. Building the infrastructure to support commercial importation would cost a tremendous amount of money and require significant changes in the law. Consequently, the savings to consumers would be less than 1 percent of total spending, while intermediaries would probably capture any other savings.

The public expectation that imported drugs are less expensive than American drugs is generally not true; example: the prices of generic drugs in other countries are on average 50 percent more than prices that Americans pay for the same generic drugs.

Six, legalized importation would most likely reduce the future development of new drugs for American consumers. It is no secret that pharmaceutical research and development spending may drop. This would result in fewer new drugs at a higher cost to Americans' health and well-being.

Seven, the effects of importation on intellectual property rights are also likely to be significant, and finally, the task force concluded that importation raises new liability concerns for consumers, manufacturers, distributors, pharmacies and other entities.

In closing, I want to state that like you, I truly appreciate the critical role of prescription drugs in our public health system. Science has brought us medications that can reduce the risk of heart attack and stroke, lower blood pressure, cure infection and save and enhance life. We must find more ways to provide these life-saving medicines to those who need them. This is being addressed, in part, through the Medicare Modernization Act and the new Medicare drug discount card.

Today, millions more seniors have access to the drugs they need, and when the Medicare Modernization Act is fully implemented less than a year from now, more seniors will have even more access to the benefits provided by the new law. There are other ways for consumers to save money on prescription drugs. Over the past few years, the FDA has worked hard to speed generic drug approvals and availability, and consumers are being encouraged to comparison shop and to ask their doctor or pharmacist for money-saving generic alternatives.

Mr. Chairman, this concludes my oral statement. I would ask that you accept my full written statement for the record. Thank you, and of course, I would be happy to answer any questions.

The CHAIRMAN. Your full written statement will be a part of the record. We will be encouraging everybody to look at the report as well as your full statement, and I appreciate the excellent summary that you have given, and I particularly was impressed with the number of hearings and people that you talked to, so our hearing is just kind of a summing down of all of the work that you did before, and of course, something gets lost in the translation every time there is one of those reductions in information, but I do appreciate all of the effort that you have gone to and the way that you presented it to us.

You suggest that personal importation is not feasible because of the volume of packages that would need to be inspected, and I assume that this is something that you presented, too, showing the numerous pictures here of the volume that are being inspected, and it assumes that we would expect the FDA to inspect every package.

What if we gave the FDA the authority to approve domestic and foreign Internet pharmacies and gave consumers the information they needed to know that these pharmacies has been approved by the FDA and that the buyer should beware of the rest of the Internet and possible hacking into the Internet? Would that be a viable way to address the safety concerns without expecting the FDA to inspect every package that comes through the mail?

Dr. CARMONA. Well, sir, I think that the premise you raise is an interesting one, but whatever Congress choses to consider as a program of importation, we would need to still make sure that the Internet pharmacies were regulated; that there was a pedigree established for each and every medication from the time of its production to the time it reaches that pharmacy and to the time it is distributed so that the patient at the other end can be certainly assured that the medication that they have is truly safe and effective and not one of the adulterated medications that we have seen so much of like in the pictures that you have seen here at the JFK center.

So certainly, Internet is one of the many options that could be considered if Congress decides to go on that path. I would just suggest that there still needs to be a process in place to ensure everything from the manufacturing to the distribution, a so-called pedigree that is established, so that every citizen is sure that they have a safe medication when they get it.

The CHAIRMAN. Thank you. Leaving the safety of the Internet and moving to the promise of anticounterfeiting technology to help ensure the safety and authenticity of prescription drugs, while this technology sounds promising, until it is universally adopted, I do not think it can be relied upon to secure safety, efficacy and integrity of the global market to safely import prescription drugs.

I am concerned that the potential cost of keeping such technology current would raise the cost of imported medicines to the point where they really would not be cost-saving to the consumers. Could you tell me anything about the cost of those technologies and how often they might have to be changed in order to stay ahead of the counterfeiter?

Dr. CARMONA. Yes, sir, in our committee, we actually asked experts to come forward and give us information on what the state-of-the-art was for so-called track and trace technology, like RFID, the radio frequency ID just being one example. In the United States now, there is considerable research going on in this area, and in some areas, there are tests going on to determine just how effective these types of technology are.

But as you implied in your question to me, this is a global issue, and we are far ahead of many other countries in this area. So for us to be able to use that effectively and partner with other countries for importation or reimportation, they would have to also engage in this technology, and we would have to have once again a method for tracking and tracing every single medication.

The costs are very difficult to estimate. We did ask the experts during the hearing. Obviously, technology development and application is expensive. Experts have told us that once in place, this technology would have to be changed fairly frequently or modified, because the fact is that there will be others out there who will figure out the system and be able to circumvent the processes we put in place.

So as with many technologies that are used to protect the consumer, we have to stay one step ahead, I mean, just like our engravers do at the Mint with the dollar bill; you know, every so often, they have to change colors and holograms and so on, because there are those that figure out the process and use it against us.

The CHAIRMAN. Thank you. As your report noted, allowing the importation of patented pharmaceuticals would impact the intellectual property rights of the developers of pharmaceutical products. I am concerned that this would result in a reduction in research and development spent on pharmaceuticals. Has HHS determined whether the incentives to invest in R&D would be diminished by legalizing drug importation? Can you discuss the impact of a reduction in R&D on pharmaceutical innovation and how that, in turn, could impact America's access to pharmaceuticals?

Dr. CARMONA. Yes, sir, these are some of the questions that we posed to the experts who came before us. The task force, being very diverse and certainly having knowledge in some of these areas, none of us really had the broader expertise that would be required. So we actively sought out experts to come and talk to us about these issues, property rights, intellectual property rights, patent rights and so on.

There is a concern that certainly, any importation program could have the potential effect of eroding research and development in this country by disincentivizing, if you will, those who invest in this very robust market. We heard time and time again how the United States is the economic pharmaceutical engine for the world, the research engine for the world. You know, we were very careful to ask questions as to what would be the short and long term consequences of any importation.

We heard time and time again from economists as well as scientists, you must be careful if you go down that path, because there is a chance that in the long run, you may undermine this very robust industry because people will not be willing to invest as they have now.

The CHAIRMAN. Thank you. My time has expired.

Senator Kennedy.

Senator KENNEDY. Thank you very much.

Of course, those companies are still making a substantial profit, even when they sell it at a cheaper price abroad. You make an extraordinarily compelling case, which I think all of us agree with, and that is that an unregulated black market system has all kinds of dangers for the American consumer. We all agree with that. That is not what we are talking about in the legislation that we have introduced. The former head of the FDA has testified, Mark McClellan, that you can get safe prescription drugs in a Canadian pharmacy.

Dr. CARMONA. Yes, sir.

Senator KENNEDY. We reviewed, when we passed the FDA legislation in 1997, what different countries in Western Europe and other countries around the world do to regulate drugs. The Canadians have a first rate system that is respected, as Mark McClellan, the former head of FDA, said. Now, if they have a sound system, why can we not find a regulated system like those tried in Massachusetts or Minnesota or Illinois and make importation from Canada safe?

Dr. CARMONA. Senator, thank you for your question.

We do agree, and I agree with my colleague Mark McClellan that the Canadian system, that part which is regulated, in fact, meets standards much like our own, that Canadian citizens can rest assured that the medications they get from their regulated pharmacies are good. What we found, though, Senator, is that when we looked at the data from Customs and Border Protection and others, we went and visited the JFK facility, that there are many out there that are purporting to be Canadian pharmacies. In fact, we found hundreds of Web sites purporting to be Canadian pharmacies when really, they were offshore gimmicks that were perpetrated on the public.

In fact, we saw some with FDA seals of approval on them which we had no knowledge of. When we went to the JFK facility, and you have some of the pictures there, we saw hundreds and hundreds of packages that come in on a daily basis, some of them Internet, some of them mail, but all of them that we saw were dangerous, because they were improperly stored, they were improperly transported, they were knockoffs; in fact, fakes, in some cases, using what looked to be a normal American label but in fact the medication inside was not that.

Senator KENNEDY. Well, are we talking then about a technology to identify for consumers the legitimate licensed Canadian Internet pharmacies?

Dr. CARMONA. Yes, sir, that is actually one of the things that we would recommend, that if Congress chooses to go down that path that we should certainly define the system. It should stay a closed system, one that is very well defined by you all, and then have the appropriate technology in place to ensure the pedigree of any medication.

Senator KENNEDY. Well, I think that is certainly what our legislation does, but what is your reaction to—I know the task force reaction—what happens in Europe with the kinds of reimportation programs that they have there and that apparently have demonstrated safety and have also had impact in terms of savings for consumers.

Dr. CARMONA. In some of the areas that we looked at, you are right, Senator, that when there is trade that is clearly regulated and standardized in pharmaceuticals, it can be done safely. As you say, some of the EU countries have demonstrated that. However, the standard that we have established in the United States for safety and pedigree establishment often exceeds what has been done in the EU, so yes, it can be done, and we fully support that.

My input to Congress would be any program that you would be willing to entertain that first should be closed. It should be well-defined. We should know every single point of entry and transport of those medications, manufacture, and it should be regulated to the highest standards, which really, our FDA has established for the world.

Senator KENNEDY. Well, I agree with you, and that is why I hope, Mr. Chairman, we are going to be able to make some progress on this, because that is certainly what we have attempted to do with our legislation, the bipartisan bill S. 334. There is the question whether the European situation is quite the same as ours, but, of course, they have different languages, so they need different labels. They still have an outstanding record of safety. We are going to hear more about it.

I think we are going to hear later about these programs, both in Minnesota and in my own State, Springfield, that have had very considerable success. My own sense is that if you have ideas, we want to work with you as a result of that task force to assure that we get the best in terms of safety. You have done a good deal of research in this area. I think you have outlined the kind of gold standard of what is necessary in terms of safety, and we will certainly want to work with you in the development of our legislation if there can be improvement.

I think in another hearing one of my colleagues, Senator Clinton, asked whether you had had a chance to review our legislation, but I think I will hold on asking you about that. I will submit some other questions just on generics, and I appreciate your presence here.

My time is up, Mr. Chairman.

The CHAIRMAN. We can easily do another round here——

Senator KENNEDY. Okay.

The CHAIRMAN. Because—

[Laughter.]

Senator KENNEDY. I like your style.

The CHAIRMAN. We do not have a lot of people waiting to ask questions.

[Laughter.]

Which really surprises me, because there has been so much attention to this. I am not sure whether they feel that they have the answers due to the completeness of the report that you did or whether there is some other reason that we do not have more people at the hearing.

On Monday, I was on CNBC briefly for—I think that was my fourth national appearance in my 8 years of being here.

[Laughter.]

I am a little reluctant to do that sort of thing, but the program started off with a Canadian minister talking about what is about to happen to their market, and he said that they only have 40 million people up there and not all of those are using prescriptions, and those are coming largely from the United States. He knew that the United States had 240 million people, and he hoped that our request for pharmaceuticals out of his country did not swamp them so bad that they could not have any.

I was listening to some of the detriments that he pointed out that we would encounter trying to go through their market to get things for our market. One of the things I am going to be doing and have started already doing as Chairman is to sit down with various groups, the doctors, other providers, the lawyers, the insurance companies, the pharmaceutical companies and even in so far as possible, the customers, which are the patients.

What I have been asking each of them is what can you do to increase access, provide more quality and keep the cost down? Of course, the first reaction by everybody is to say what the lawyers can do or what the insurance company can do and what the doctors can do. No, no, that is not what we are trying to do here. I want to know what you can do to hold down the costs, to increase quality and access.

Once they start thinking about it, I am really pleased with the ideas that people have come up with for ways that they can participate, and I think that may provide us with some solutions on all of this. On pharmaceuticals, it seems a little convoluted to me to have to go through Canada or any other country to get lower-cost pharmaceuticals, and I did note the concern of the Canadian minister.

Getting back to the questions here, in order to truly implement safe importation, pending proposals rely on this pedigree that you have mentioned several times or paperwork that can accompany the drugs from the foreign suppliers to the exporters in this country. Now, counterfeiters are able to copy packaging, the holograms, security mechanisms, the shape of the pill, the kind of the bottle. We have had the FDA testify before on kinds of problems that they see.

Now, in terms of working with other countries in the context of this commercial importation, how would we ensure the authenticity of these paper pedigrees and verify that it is indeed an authentic document and not something made on somebody's computer or at the local Kinko's? Would other countries have to agree to assure the accuracy of those pedigrees, or would those kinds of arrangements have to be in place prior to implementation and then change fairly frequently?

So what have you learned about the willingness of other countries to do this?

Dr. CARMONA. We reached out, Senator, to any and all countries who would weigh in on this, and really, Switzerland and Canada were our big takers. There were not a lot of people interested, because they recognized, we heard, the cost of developing such a system: you are right in that looking at the global marketplace, whoever we decided to partner with would have to embrace the same technology, because what we would be doing is interconnectiveness in a newly-established system, whichever country we were working with.

It really goes far beyond paper. What we are really talking is more advanced technology, which is electronic. There really does not have to be movement of paper. Tracking and tracing technology can be done all electronically. But you still have to stay a step ahead of your adversaries, who are always going to be looking to figure out a way to make that hologram the same way you do or the watermark in the medication or somehow get themselves into our system so that they can, you know, potentially put counterfeit medications in there.

So we are concerned about that. But the underlying premise is true: we would have to form partnerships, and other countries who would want to engage in this type of trade with us would have to fully embrace this technology and the philosophy of the system that we are creating, yes, sir.

The CHAIRMAN. Thank you, now, my understanding is that the European Union does not allow importation from outside its borders; is that correct?

Dr. CARMONA. Generally speaking, sir, the European Union acts much like our States do. There is State regulation, and they have relationships between countries that are still blossoming in the new EU, but in general, that is correct.

The CHAIRMAN. Okay, thank you, and one more very quick question: you mentioned that the FDA seal of approval is being used on some Web sites that definitely are not approved by the FDA. Is there any kind of international enforcement against that, and where would that take place?

Dr. CARMONA. Well, it is very limited, sir, and that is why some of the folks that we found that were doing these things are very clever. They will put a Web site up in Canada and have a name that implies they are a Canadian-sanctioned organization, which lets people believe, oh, Canada has similar standards to the United States; then, it must be safe.

The fact is that the Canadian Government has told us repeatedly they do not regulate those sites. They regulate the pharmaceuticals in Canada for use by their citizens. So anybody can come, spend $50, put a Web site up, and what we have found, our investigators have found, that often, the billing is offshore someplace. The drug is being made in some country far, far away from here, not in Canada. Canada is used as a passthrough so that they can call it a Canadian drug, and the bottom line is the public gets something that we have no idea if it is safe or effective or could even be harmful to the public.

We have seen that quite often, both at the JFK Center as well as the Internet sites that our staff, FDA and DEA and Customs and Border Protection have investigated.

The CHAIRMAN. Thank you. My time has expired again.

Senator Kennedy.

Senator KENNEDY. Just quickly, did you examine any of the existing city or State import programs in terms of safety? Did you look at any of those States?

Dr. CARMONA. Senator, we did not look at them specifically. We did have some of the governors and State officials come and speak to us about their programs, but we stuck with the questions that were posed to us by Congress, and we did not go off on many of those tangents to, you know, look at if those systems were safe and effective and so on.

Senator KENNEDY. Because I have been impressed by the success, first of all, in safety. In Springfield, MA, a determination was made about a certain Canadian pharmacy that was highly regarded, and Springfield worked out the contractual arrangements with tens of thousands of dollars in savings. When FDA looked at this pharmacy, they had one bad case with insulin. Our legislation does not permit importation of insulin, in part, because of the refrigeration issues.

But other States, as I understand we will hear from Governor Pawlenty, have a Web site which identifies legitimate Canadian pharmacies. Although I suppose people can try to hack into the site to disrupt it like they can any other site—and it has worked. Illinois has used their State Board of Health, and they went up and examined the companies themselves that they were going to import from and have very much involved local pharmacies to give patients guidance, and they have had a very impressive program. Other States in that region now are joining it.

So these programs and our legislation has a way a way of proceeding that I think does about as much as you can do in terms of safety, and listening to your comments, I think, certainly, we would meet your criteria. We will, as I mentioned earlier, work with you, because I think there are a variety of different ways of doing it. I think these States, these governors, these mayors, have put safety as a first priority. Nothing is going to be 100 percent perfect in this world, but the difference that it makes in terms of prescription drugs, which are so necessary to the health of many of our seniors and others, has just been extremely dramatic, and when we are not having negotiated prices for the Medicare prescription drug benefit, as we do in the VA system, our seniors are under incredible pressure, and I think this fairly cries out for action. But again, I want to thank you and indicate that we will certainly work with you and your task force to give the highest priority to the issues of safety.

I wanted to just mention, Mr. Chairman, on the question we have for why some of our colleagues are not here. We have Secretary Rice, who just returned, appearing before the Foreign Relations Committee. Senator Dodd is over there. In EPW, on clear skies, we have Senator Jeffords and Senator Clinton. In the Banking Committee, we have Secretary Levitt in the Finance Committee and Mr. Greenspan in the Banking Committee, so there are a lot of pressures on our colleagues. I know, as you do on your side, the great interest in this issue, because this is really a bipartisan issue of great concern to our seniors and others.

The CHAIRMAN. Right, you and I will be working with the other members of the committee to come up with some solutions.

Senator Murray.

Senator MURRAY. Thank you, Mr. Chairman. I really appreciate your holding this hearing. I think it is really an important one. We do hear a lot about reimportation at home, and Dr. Carmona, thank you so much for coming and testifying on the work of your committee.

I always worry when we start talking about reimportation that we are not looking at a lot of the real issues that are facing us in terms of prescription drugs, the coverage gap with Medicare and 44 million people who are uninsured today who do not have access to any health care whatsoever. When we talk about reimportation, it is not going to deal with a number of the issues that really are impacting our health care, but it is an issue out there and one that we need to really understand what we are doing. I have always been concerned about the safety and efficacy of our drugs and want to make sure that if we move down this road, we do it correctly, so I appreciate the work that you and the task force have done.

One of the interesting findings that I saw was the degree to which consumers are already importing drugs into the United States for personal use, and I know we have had previous hearings where we have seen drugs that have come in from China and Belize with Web sites someplace else, and we have had testimony from families that have been impacted by drugs that have come in that have had devastating effects.

So we have to be careful what we do. I wanted the chance to ask you this morning, how do we protect consumers from the risks of reimportation or from purchasing on the Internet?

Dr. CARMONA. Senator, I think that our most important endeavor in this task force is the safety to our citizens, as I know it is for you. The way to do that is to make sure that whatever system Congress decides on that it is what we would define as a closed system, and closed meaning we have hundreds and hundreds of portals of entry around the country, and if you then look at each individual being able to import whenever they want, you have thousands of combinations and permutations, and we cannot guarantee safety.

A closed system would say these are the sites we can deal with, whether Internet or fixed. These are the sites that the FDA will have authority to work with and make sure that the processes are up to standard, that packaging, marketing, et cetera, transport of the medication, a pedigree is established. So I think the underlying premise is that whichever path Congress decides to take that we make sure the system is prospectively well-defined, and we can ensure the pedigree of each and every medication that comes to us from any source.

Senator MURRAY. I noticed that the task force asked for comments from foreign governments about their willingness or ability to implement new or additional protections to ensure safety. Did you get any comments from any foreign governments?

Dr. CARMONA. Senator, very few. We heard through the grapevine, if you will, that most did not want to comment. They recognized the extreme cost and some of the economic burden it may place on them to look at this kind of trade. We did hear from Canada, of course, because that was the driving force. We heard also from Switzerland, but very limited remarks in this area.

But we feel, though, strongly that any partnerships that were created, that the partner would really have to embrace the technology and the concept of pedigree to ensure safety on both sides.

Senator MURRAY. Can we assume that Canada has the same drug approval and safety standards that we do or not?

Dr. CARMONA. According to our FDA experts, I have been told that the regulatory process in Canada is very similar and that Canadians can feel as assured as Americans in purchasing drugs from Canadian-regulated pharmacies with licensed pharmacists, pretty much an analogous situation to the United States.

Senator MURRAY. Now, I know that the task force was instructed to evaluate the safety and security of the U.S. drug supply. But we have seen evidence that some large purchasers in the United States like the VA or Medicaid programs get big discounts today when they do negotiation. Is there any concern that importation would eliminate any of those discounts that we currently have for Medicaid or for VA?

Dr. CARMONA. Senator, I would only be able to give you a guess at that. That is not something we studied within the task force.

Senator MURRAY. So you did not look at that at all. Okay, all right.

Well, I think that we have a real challenge in front of us. I think people are crying out for lower drug costs. We have to find a way to get there. But I think one of the things we really have to work very hard at as policy makers is to make sure we do it safely and effectively and in a way that American consumers know that their families are safe when they purchase drugs. So I appreciate the work of the task force.

Thank you.

Dr. CARMONA. Thank you, ma'am.

The CHAIRMAN. Thank you for your great addition to the record.

Dr. Carmona, I thank you for being here. I thank you for all of the effort you put into the task force. I am not sure we have had a Surgeon General that has had quite as diverse a background as you do, which really contributes to information and decisions that you make and pass on to us. I am not sure we have had a Surgeon General before who was in the Army before they went to college or that served as a paramedic and a nurse as well as a doctor. So we thank you for that diverse background and the way that that leads to good decisions.

Thank you for your testimony. We will leave the record open so that perhaps some other questions can be asked yet to build the record a little bit more fully. Thank you.

Dr. CARMONA. Thank you, Mr. Chairman; thank you, Senators.

[The prepared statement of Dr. Carmona follows:]

PREPARED STATEMENT OF RICHARD H. CARMONA

INTRODUCTION

Good morning Mr. Chairman and distinguished members of the committee. My name is Dr. Richard Carmona, and I am the Surgeon General of the United States Public Health Service. I appreciate having this opportunity to discuss the work of the HHS Task Force on Drug Importation and issues relating to the importation of prescription drugs into the United States.

BRIEF OVERVIEW OF DRUG IMPORTATION

The Federal Food, Drug, and Cosmetic (FD&C) Act limits the types of drugs that may be imported into the United States. Currently, the only types of legally imported drugs are: (1) those that are manufactured in foreign FDA-inspected facilities and the subject of an FDA-approved drug application, or (2) those that are U.S.-approved and manufactured in the United States, sent abroad, then re-imported to the United States by the manufacturer under proper controls and in compliance with FD&C Act requirements.

All imported drugs are required to meet the same standards as domestic drugs, and thus cannot be unapproved, misbranded, or adulterated. The FD&C Act prohibits individuals from importing unapproved, misbranded, or adulterated drugs into the United States. This prohibition extends to drugs that are foreign versions of U.S.-approved medications, and drugs dispensed without a prescription.

Although importing unapproved prescription drugs is illegal, FDA may exercise its enforcement discretion and not take action against illegal personal importation in certain situations. FDA has developed a policy to guide its exercise of enforcement discretion with respect to importation of the products it regulates. This policy is called the personal importation policy, and it was last updated in 1988 in response to concerns that certain AIDS treatments were not available in the United

States. Under the policy, FDA exercises its enforcement discretion under certain circumstances and does not stop individuals with serious conditions from bringing into the United States treatments that are legally available in foreign countries but are not approved in the United States.

THE MEDICARE PRESCRIPTION DRUG, IMPROVEMENT AND MODERNIZATION ACT OF 2003 (MMA)

In 2003, Congress passed the Medicare Prescription Drug, Improvement and Modernization Act of 2003 (Medicare Modernization Act or MMA), which provides an important new prescription drug benefit for seniors. MMA also includes provisions aimed at providing lower cost drugs to consumers.

MMA provides authority for pharmacists and wholesalers to import certain drugs from Canada, subject to certain conditions. The drug importation provisions in MMA only become effective if the Secretary of HHS first certifies that implementing the program will pose no additional risk to public health and safety and will result in a significant reduction in the cost of such drugs to the American consumer. In addition, MMA directs the Secretary of HHS to grant waivers to permit importation of a 90-day supply of any FDA-approved prescription drug imported from Canada from a licensed pharmacy for personal use.

MMA also required the Secretary of HHS to complete a comprehensive study that identifies problems with implementation of existing law and examines a range of issues associated with the importation of drugs.

HHS TASK FORCE ON DRUG IMPORTATION

On February 26, 2004, then-HHS Secretary Tommy G. Thompson announced the creation of a task force to advise him on how to address the drug importation questions posed by Congress in the Medicare Modernization Act. I served as the chairman of the task force, which was comprised of 13 senior executives with diverse experience from across the Federal Government.

The Task Force was charged with gathering input, ideas, and expertise from the public on issues related to drug importation. One of the main goals of the Task Force was to ensure an open and transparent process that provided an opportunity for all views to be heard. To that end, the Task Force held six listening sessions, including an open public meeting, heard from more than 100 presenters and received information from over 100 individuals and organizations via the Task Force's online docket.

Among the presenters were consumer representatives, pharmaceutical industry representatives, international regulatory and industry representatives, academicians, health care purchasers, professional medical groups, government and elected officials, and members of the public.

In addition, a group of Task Force members conducted a site visit to John F. Kennedy International Airport in New York City to see how imported drugs are processed daily by U.S. Customs and Border Protection (CBP) and Food and Drug Administration (FDA) officials. This site visit demonstrated to us the huge challenge of ensuring the safety of imported drugs.

REPORT ON PRESCRIPTION DRUG IMPORTATION

The Task Force produced a report that contains our findings based on all of the information presented to us and expert views solicited from appropriate government agencies. The report is available online at *http://www.hhs.gov/importtaskforce/*. The key findings of the Task Force are:

1. The current system of drug regulation in the United States has been very effective in protecting public safety, but is facing new threats. It should be modified only with great care to ensure continued high standards of safety and effectiveness for the U.S. drug supply.

• Safety and protection of the public health are paramount; safety should not be sacrificed for affordability.

• There are particular products of concern, including controlled substances, intravenous products, biologics, drugs that must be refrigerated or frozen, drugs that have specific post-marketing risk management programs, drugs that are highly susceptible to counterfeiting on the global market, and those that have less expensive alternatives (i.e., generics) in the United States, that pose special concerns in the importation context.

• To maintain current levels of safety, standards of practice at the level that currently exist in the United States would need to apply to all foreign drug suppliers under a commercial importation program. In addition, Memoranda of Understanding (MOU) may be needed with the affected countries to ensure effective enforcement.

• There are promising new and emerging anti-counterfeiting technologies; however, until they are universally adopted, they cannot be adequately relied upon to secure the safety, efficacy, and integrity of the global market to safely import prescription drugs into the United States.

2. There are significant risks associated with the way individuals are currently importing drugs that violate the FD&C Act.

• According to CBP, there are 355 "points of entry" for access into the United States. This includes 14 international mail branches, 29 express consignment facilities, and 312 ports. Given the broad responsibilities assigned to FDA, only a limited number of FDA inspectors are available to staff the 14 international mail facilities in the United States that receive millions of small packages a year, where they historically have had to inspect only a small number of large commercial pharmaceutical imports.

• FDA currently does not have sufficient resources to ensure adequate inspection of current levels of personal shipments of prescription drugs entering the United States. Moreover, to maintain an adequate inspection of current levels of commercially imported pharmaceutical products would require significant investment in information technology and personnel, among other things.

• Imported drugs are arriving from all corners of the world, including developed and emerging countries. Nearly 5 million shipments, comprising about 12 million prescription drug products with a value of approximately $700 million, entered the United States from Canada alone in 2003. The report estimates that an equivalent amount of prescription drugs may come in from the rest of the world.

• Many state-licensed Internet pharmacies provide a legitimate means for consumers to access safe and effective medicines, but others raise significant safety concerns. Some sellers of imported drugs are "rogue" Internet pharmacies that pretend to be legitimate and operate behind facades. Many of the drugs sold over the Internet claim to be interchangeable with the approved U.S. drug, but are not.

• Purchasing prescription drugs over the Internet without a prescription has been found to be relatively easy to accomplish. In those cases, the lack of an adequate health professional/patient relationship is of particular concern.

3. It would be extraordinarily difficult and costly for "personal" importation to be implemented in a way that ensures the safety and effectiveness of the imported drugs.

• There is no realistic level of resources that could ensure that personally imported drugs are adequately inspected to assure their safety since visual inspection, testing, and oversight of all personally imported prescription drugs are not feasible or practical at this time.

• The report estimates that 10 million packages containing prescription drugs entered the United States in 2003. It is estimated that it would cost $3 billion to examine all of these packages.

4. Overall national savings from legalized commercial importation will likely be a small percentage of total drug spending and developing and implementing such a program would incur significant costs and require significant additional authorities.

• A commercial importation program could be feasible but would require new legal authorities, substantial additional resources, and significant restrictions on the type of drugs that could be imported, which could increase the costs of imported drugs.

• Total savings to drug buyers from legalized commercial importation would be 1 to 2 percent of total drug spending and much less than international price comparisons might suggest. The savings going directly to individuals would be less than 1 percent of total spending. Most of the savings would likely go to third party payers, such as insurance companies and HMOs.

• Under legalized importation, intermediaries may capture a large part of the potential savings.

5. The public expectation that most imported drugs are less expensive than American drugs is not generally true.

• The prices foreigners pay for generic drugs are on average 50 percent greater than prices Americans pay for generic drugs.

• There is evidence that greater use of U.S.-approved generic drugs by Americans could reduce drug spending by billions of dollars annually.

• Foreign drug supplies in many countries that might export to the United States are sufficiently small relative to U.S. drug consumption as to raise questions about the sustainability of high-volume exports from those countries.

• To the extent that prescription drugs are eligible for importation from the same company at a lower price than in the United States, potential quantity constraints imposed by manufacturers or foreign governments would limit the eligible supply and the benefits to U.S. consumers.

6. Legalized importation will likely adversely affect the future development of new drugs for American consumers.

• Americans have a greater choice of newly launched pharmaceutical products than foreigners. In recent years, more than 40 percent of new drugs were launched first in the United States.

• Under a legalized commercial importation program, R&D spending would drop, which could result in between 4 to 18 fewer new drugs introduced per decade, at a substantial cost to society.

• Estimates of reduced benefits, due to reduced R&D spending, to future drug consumers may range from $5 billion to $20 billion per decade without including gains from having a greater variety of generics in the future. Reduced benefits may significantly offset savings from legalized importation.

7. The effects of legalized importation on intellectual property rights are uncertain but likely to be significant.

• Importation could impact the intellectual property rights of developers of pharmaceutical products and could be subject to challenge under domestic law, including possibly the U.S. Constitution, and international intellectual property rules.

• It is likely that intellectual property rights holders will exercise their rights to the fullest extent available under the law and the effects may impact the availability of imported drugs.

• International agreements recognizing intellectual property rights may be affected by the legalization of importation.

8. Legalized importation raises liability concerns for consumers, manufacturers, distributors, pharmacies, and other entities.

• Allowing prescription drug importation would have uncertain effects on the litigation exposure of manufacturers, distributors, doctors, and pharmacists.

• To deal with these risks, entities in the pharmaceutical distribution chain would likely take additional costly defensive actions.

• Some potentially liable parties could be unavailable to U.S. courts and, therefore, to consumers, industry, or health care providers.

CONCLUSION

As a trauma surgeon, the former CEO of a health system, and now doctor to the American people, I understand the critical role that prescription drugs have in our public health system. It is truly wonderful that science has brought us medications that can reduce the risk of heart attack and stroke, lower blood pressure, cure infection, and save and enhance life. As a society we must find more ways to provide these life-saving medicines to those who need them.

President Bush and Secretary Thompson, as well as my task force colleague Dr. McClellan, have already made great strides with the initial implementation of the Medicare Modernization Act and the new Medicare drug discount card. Today, millions more seniors are getting access to the drugs that they need, and as the Medicare Modernization Act becomes fully implemented in the coming years, even more seniors will have even more access to the preventative and drug benefits provided through the new law.

In addition to the new Medicare drug discount card, there are other ways for U.S. consumers to save money on domestic prescription drugs. Consumers are encouraged to shop around for price comparisons, ask their doctor or pharmacist for generic alternatives, and take advantage of prescription drug discount cards.

Thank you. I will be happy to answer any questions you may have.

The CHAIRMAN. Can we have the next panel move up to the table, please? See if we can have the Governor on this side, followed by—it would be the Honorable Tim Pawlenty, the Governor of Minnesota, from St. Paul, MN; then, Mr. John Gray, president and CEO of the Healthcare Distribution Management Association in Reston, VA; then, Mr. Carmen Catizone, the executive director of the National Association of Boards of Pharmacy, from Mount Prospect, IL; and Dr. Peter Rost, the vice-president of Marketing for Endocrine Care of Pfizer.

I want to thank all of you for serving on this panel. We know that it will greatly enhance our knowledge of drug reimportation, both the realities of the safety and the security. We appreciate the experience that each of you have had in that area. Again, I will ask each of you to summarize your testimony. Your full testimony will be part of the record but if you can do a summary, that would allow us more opportunity for questions.

Begin with Governor Pawlenty.

STATEMENT OF HON. TIM PAWLENTY, GOVERNOR OF THE STATE OF MINNESOTA, ST. PAUL, MN

Governor PAWLENTY. Good morning, Mr. Chairman, Senator Kennedy, members of the committee, thank you for the chance to be here and share a few thoughts about the Minnesota experience. Senator Kennedy, Springfield, MA, of course was the pioneer in this area, and Minnesota was the first State to do it, and we have got some pioneers there including Senator Dayton and Congressman Gutknecht and others who have helped with our effort and helped blaze the trail.

In short, I think the American health care delivery system is broken. I think there are many observers who believe it is going to collapse in the next 15 to 20 years for a whole variety of reasons. The lack of affordability of prescription medicines is one reason, one of the forces or factors that is contributing to that challenge and I think a burgeoning crisis. One troubling aspect, of course, is we have too many Americans who, for a variety of reasons cannot afford or cannot access affordable prescription medicines.

Downstairs in this building, when you enter the Dirksen Senate Office Building at one of the entrances is a tribute to Senator Dirksen. It honors him for, quote, "his unerring sense of the possible." We have before us today a chance to make progress on one piece of a critically important issue for a lot of Americans and certainly a lot of Minnesotans, and that is access to affordable prescription medicines.

Mr. Chair and Senators, what you hear in this debate and see a lot in this debate is the dangling of the shiny object. You see folks who distract from what is actually happening or what is proposed in legislation to draw your attention to other concerns or aspects. Senator Kennedy, I think you hit it right on the nail when you said earlier that we are not proposing to go out and encourage people to use rogue Internet pharmacies or encourage people to access counterfeiters. If you go to licensed, established, credible, reputable Canadian pharmacies, there is no evidence, I repeat there is no evidence that as applied to those pharmacies, those operations that the safety concerns exist in any manner.

So, what you see in the debate is advocates, the opponents who come forward with the shiny object and say there are Indonesian operations; there are Middle Eastern operations; they counterfeit; they mislabel; they change the doses; they do all sorts of nasty things. Well, that is all very interesting, but that is not what we are proposing. We are proposing, ideally, the Federal Government but at the very least State governments use their regulatory and health and safety powers to step forward and identify for consumers in a credible, reliable way the licensed, established, credible operations that can provide these medicines at a discount to Minnesotans and to American consumers, and if we do it that way, as is the focus of your legislation, there is not a problem.

Then, the question becomes one of logistics. In Minnesota, MN, like in every other State in the country, we have a large veterans hospital. Every day, every week, they mail out hundreds, thousands of pharmacy prescription medicines. It is done safely, and so, the premise being that they can do it from Minneapolis, but you cannot mail or FedEx or UPS a prescription from Winnipeg to Duluth? I just do not buy it, Mr. Chairman. Neither do the consumers who are using our service.

In short, what we have is two Web sites, one for all consumers in Minnesota, one for our State employees. They go on the Web site. They have to have a prescription from their own doctor. They download an order form. They send it up to the pharmacy in Canada. It is countersigned by a Canadian doctor. We have gone up, inspected, contracted with these Canadian pharmacies to meet our protocols. They have done that.

We have over 9,000 prescriptions who have been fulfilled through this process, and you know what the number one complaint is in this process? Our own Federal Government. Our number one complaint is the FDA or the Postal Service or the Customs agency has interfered and disrupted the delivery of the drugs or delayed the service. We have had no, zero, none, safety complaints or incidents with respect to our program.

I think you are well aware of the arguments for and against. I will not belabor the point and will invite your questions, but I just encourage you as this debate unfolds to not avert your gaze to the shiny object, which is the horrible things that we all admit happen on the Internet. It is full of bad characters, shady characters and the like, but that is not what we are proposing. We are asking the government, ideally the FDA, the ones who are best suited, well suited, equipped, have specialty and expertise to step in and identify the credible, reputable operators in Canada or elsewhere, and then, it is just a matter of trusting, like we do every day through our American mail order pharmacies, that we have the logistics and distribution systems to deliver the medicine. We have done it.

So in closing, I would just say if Congress cannot or will not or is unable to act, please at least follow the advice of Paul McCartney when he sang, Let It Be.

[Laughter.]

If you cannot help us, please stay out of the way, and let it be so that we can continue to demonstrate that this can work. Eventually, we will mount enough evidence where it will become obvious and compelling. So, help us if you can, but in the worst case, please let it be. Thank you.

[The prepared statement of Governor Pawlenty follows:]

PREPARED STATEMENT OF GOVERNOR TIM PAWLENTY, GOVERNOR OF ST. PAUL, MN

Chairman Enzi, Senator Kennedy, and members of the Senate Committee on Health, Education, Labor, and Pensions, it is an honor to be with you today.

As I entered this building this morning, I saw the tribute to Senator Everett Dirksen carved in the marble downstairs. It strikes a fitting tone for his hearing.

It honored Senator Dirksen for "his unerring sense of the possible that enabled him to know when to compromise; by such men are our freedoms retained."

In an increasingly polarized environment, we need to know when to compromise and practice the art of the possible.

If ever there was an issue that we can come together on this is it. The rising cost of prescription drugs has sparked a prairie fire that is spreading across our Nation. Today we have an opportunity to make bold steps toward progress.

We've all heard the arguments about why Americans pay more for prescription drugs than other countries. But the bottom line is that Americans pay more than the rest of the world and the price differential puts prescription medicines out of reach for too many Americans. The current situation is unfair and untenable.

That's why in Minnesota we've decided to take action. We're taking a method, trying it and finding strong success.

MINNESOTA'S PLAN

The Minnesota Plan for Prescription Drugs has a very simple goal—to get a better deal for Minnesotans. We have established a program to facilitate the purchase of prescription drugs from Canada by individuals.

We have established two Web sites—MinnesotaRxConnect.com for all Minnesota citizens and Advantage-Meds.com for State employees, retirees and their dependents.

Through MinnesotaRxConnect, Minnesotans are able to determine if their prescription medications are available at a lower cost from a Canadian pharmacy, and if so, how to order them. The site focuses on maintenance drugs that can be shipped safely from Canada. Only reputable Canadian pharmacies licensed by a Canadian province, willing to have their facilities and safety protocols reviewed by the Minnesota Department of Human Services are used. The four pharmacies affiliated with MinnesotaRxConnect have each been visited by pharmacists employed by the State of Minnesota, including Minnesota Board of Pharmacy inspectors. The site also lets consumers know if there is a lower cost generic alternative about which they should see their doctor.

In addition, MinnesotaRxConnect is about more than just Canadian importation. It provides tips about how to become an informed consumer of prescription medicines including links to other programs that might assist consumers in purchasing their medications, such as State and pharmaceutical manufacturer programs.

Those individuals wishing to take advantage of the program need to obtain a prescription from their own physician and send a copy of the prescription, an order form and a medical history questionnaire to the Canadian pharmacy. To comply with Canadian law, the prescription is reviewed and countersigned by a Canadian physician. Assuming that all is in order, the pharmacy ships the medication to the patient by mail in the manufacturer's original, sealed container whenever possible.

Since the launch of MinnesotaRxConnect a little over 1 year ago, the Canadian pharmacies have filled more than 9,000 prescriptions for people ordering through the site. We have received only a couple of complaints about the pharmacies regarding billing issues. Those complaints were quickly resolved by the pharmacies when the State contacted them. We have received no complaints about the quality, effectiveness or safety of the drugs.

Let me repeat—we have not received a single complaint, out of more than 9,000 prescriptions filled—regarding the quality, effectiveness or safety of the drugs that were purchased utilizing our prescription drug Web site.

The top complaint we have received is not regarding Canadian pharmacies or drugs, but about enforcement actions taken by the U.S. Government. A number of packages shipped by the pharmacies affiliated with our Web sites have been seized by the FDA, Customs or the Postal Service. When notified, the pharmacies promptly ship another supply at no cost to the customer.

Consumers who use MinnesotaRxConnect must first visit with their personal physician and get a prescription from them. The prescription is reviewed by Canadian pharmacists who contact the U.S. physician to clear up any potential problems. The prescription and the patient's medical history are then sent to the Canadian physician for yet another review. A Canadian physician then countersigns the prescription.

Recently, the Canadian government has raised concerns about the practice of countersigning. Canada's Minister of Health has said he considers physician countersigning to be unethical. We disagree. We see the countersigning process as an additional safety check, one more opportunity for a medical professional to review the prescription for potential problems.

If the Canadian physician was the only doctor involved, it would be unethical for them to issue a prescription to someone they had never seen or examined. But in this process, the Canadian physician is only double-checking a process that first included the patient being examined by their doctor and that doctor issuing a prescription.

Unfortunately, there are some unethical web-based operations that will have a physician write prescriptions based only on an online questionnaire that the patient fills out. In such cases, no physician sees the patient. Our system ensures that this does not happen by requiring that the patient meet with and receive a prescription from their physician.

Through a second Web site, Advantage-Meds.com, State employees, retirees and their dependents can purchase certain prescription medicines at no cost through one of the Canadian mail order pharmacies affiliated with MinnesotaRxConnect.

During 2004 (May 13—Dec 31):

1. 1,861 members enrolled.
   - Eligible members include 48,000 employees and 72,000 dependents;
   - A member can enroll but not order a drug;
   - A member can order more than one drug.
2. 3,166 drugs were ordered.
   - An order is one 3-month supply of one drug;
   - Represents about 1 percent of the drugs purchased by members.
3. 27,526 persons made 42,232 visits to the Web site.
4. $577,479 was spent by program.
   - Average of $76,992 per month (7.5 months);
   - Average cost of $184 per drug (3 month order).
5. Approximately $300,000 was saved by program and members.
   - $98 per drug;
     - $53 to program in reduced costs;
     - $45 to members in waived co-payments;
   - Results meet initial expectations.

We recognize that these measures are not the long-term solution. They are, however, designed to provide short-term relief and to build pressure for long-term reform.

ENSURING SAFETY

Those who oppose reimportation often talk of great problems with safety. On this point, it is important to be clear about what we have done.

We reference services available from established, reputable, credible, accredited Canadian pharmacies. There is no evidence to suggest such pharmacies are unsafe. To the contrary, Minnesota Board of Pharmacy surveyors have visited the pharmacies and found no significant problems. Canadians are not dying or at risk because of their system. Assertions that a program like Minnesota's is unsafe suggests either the pharmacies we have chosen are unsafe or they are too inept to properly mail or deliver medicines safely. Neither is true. Moreover many reputable, established pharmacies in the United States already use a mail order, Internet or phone order system. The FDA apparently thinks it works well for them. For example, the Veterans Hospital in Minneapolis mails out a large number of prescriptions to patients each week.

Our program should not be confused with the questionable Internet pharmacy or "storefront" marketing entities that offer or have offered their services to U.S. citizens with little or no oversight. We agree that such operations present an unreasonable safety risk to consumers.

Our Department of Human Services conducted a review of Canadian practices, similar but independent of that done by the State of Illinois. We came to the same conclusion that they did: the Canadian system is comparable to ours in safety standards.

There is a misperception that reimportation from Canada is some risky endeavor in which we give up safety to use a Third World apothecary just to save a dime. Canada's pharmaceutical regulatory system is strong and effective. At the State level, we continue to monitor and ensure that those pharmacies serving our citizens are held to the highest standards of safety.

Let me briefly explain to you some of the safety and security protocols we are using as part of our reimportation program:

1. The pharmacies associated with our Web site are licensed by the Canadian province in which they are located;
2. The pharmacies have agreed to allow unannounced inspections of their facilities, and the Minnesota Department of Human Services Pharmacy Program Man-

ager, who is a pharmacist, has conducted unannounced follow-up visits to all four pharmacies;

3. Medications are dispensed in the manufacturer's unopened, safety-sealed containers in appropriate amounts whenever possible;

4. Medications shipped are approved for use in Canada by the Therapeutic Products Directorate of Health Canada, which uses standards similar to those of the FDA when approving drugs.

THE INDUSTRY'S ACTIONS

Pharmaceutical manufacturers such as Merck, Pfizer, Eli Lilly and others have withheld supplies of prescription drugs from Canadian pharmacies that serve Americans.

Their actions are unfortunate. I urge this committee to review the comments and actions of the companies involved.

MINNESOTA IS READY TO LEAD THE WAY

The States are often called the "laboratories of democracy." The State of Minnesota is proving that again by moving ahead in implementing this prescription medicine plan.

Let us be the experiment. Let us try it. Let us continue to put the arguments to the test. If it doesn't work, we'll admit it. The current system is not "safe" because too many people can't afford their medicine.

Thank you very much.

MINNESOTA RXCONNECT ONLINE

Minnesota RxConnect Online, *www.MinnesotaRxConnect.com,* was created to provide Minnesotans information on issues related to prescription medicine, safety and cost-saving tips, and programs to help low-income Minnesotans pay for prescription medications.

This site also provides Minnesotans with information about accessing lower-cost prescription medicine from Canada. The site hosts a list of medicines and prices available through four Canadian pharmacies. Consumers can print order forms from the site for individual use in placing an order with a pharmacy. (Orders cannot be placed online through the site.)

SITE ACTIVITY FROM JAN. 30TH (LAUNCH DATE) THROUGH JANUARY 2005

Total number of site visits (aka 'hits'): 174,599
Total number of prescriptions ordered: 9,006
Total cost of all prescriptions ordered: $1,119,190
Number of medications listed on the site (at launch): 821
Activity by Pharmacy

	Total Care Pharmacy	Granville Pharmacy	Canada U.S. Pharmacy	CanadaDrugs .com	Totals
New prescriptions	1,214	1,881	2,015	509	5,619
Refill prescriptions	1,198	1,018	918	253	3,387
Total prescriptions	2,412	2,899	2,933	762	9,006
Average cost of prescription	$126.38	$148.06	$136.00	$115.92	

The CHAIRMAN. Thank you for your enthusiastic and innovative testimony. We really appreciate that.

Mr. John Gray.

STATEMENT OF JOHN M. GRAY, PRESIDENT AND CEO, HEALTHCARE DISTRIBUTION MANAGEMENT ASSOCIATION (HDMA), RESTON, VA

Mr. GRAY. Thank you, Mr. Chairman, Senator Kennedy, members of the committee.

My name is John Gray. I am the president and CEO of the Healthcare Distribution Management Association, HDMA. We have worked with our members, the Nation's 46 full-service distributors to secure a safe, efficient, reliable distribution system that provides life saving health care products and services. Our member companies are responsible for the daily delivery of over 9 million of the Nation's prescription drugs to more than 130,000 retail pharmacies, hospital, nursing homes, clinics and other provider sites in all 50 States.

My purpose here is to emphasize four key points: the primary responsibility of the health care industry is to ensure patient safety and health. Our mission as a health care distributor is to ensure that the prescription drug supply chain remains safe, secure and tightly regulated. Any efforts to permit importation of prescription drugs from abroad must not weaken this system.

Significant efforts are underway and should continue to further secure our own domestic supply chain in the face of what we see as an increasing incidence of counterfeit and adulterated products entering our markets from domestic and foreign sources. There is no single solution to secure the integrity of the prescription drug supply. The only effective response is a series of multiple strategies, including participation from all participants in our supply chain here in the United States.

The Nation's drug system is highly regulated at both Federal and State levels. The Federal and State partnership has served the Nation well to date. However, even the United States now is no longer immune from the growing and increasingly sophisticated threat of counterfeiting. According to the FDA, the number of instances where counterfeit products have been breached into the domestic supply chain that have been reported to them have gone from six cases just 5 years ago to over 22 cases in the year 2003.

Given the increasing sophistication and frequency of counterfeiting, it is imperative that we remain vigilant and seek new approaches to secure the domestic prescription drug supply. The effort should include three items: strengthening government regulation, oversight and enforcement; adopting new technologies; and developing and implementing what we call best industry practices.

HDMA joined the FDA's call for States' review and revised their current wholesale licensing statutes and regulations. We have undertaken the added step of drafting our own model legislation under consideration in multiple States. This bill calls for additional requirements to be met in order to receive a prescription drug distribution license as well as increased State oversight and enforcement measures. While many States have taken the licensure and inspection responsibilities seriously, we at HDMA remain concerned that too few States have devoted sufficient attention and resources to this area.

We believe that significant variation in the levels of State regulation of pharmaceutical distributors has led to inconsistent standards being applied across the United States. We think this must change and will continue to advocate for stronger, more uniform national standards for the licensure of pharmaceutical distributors. HDMA also believes that technology can serve an important role in securing our drug supply. However, no single technology can prevent counterfeiting by itself.

We believe that deployment of electronic product codes, radio frequency ID or RFID hold the most promise for tracking and tracing and authenticating product movement across our supply chain. Using RFID technology, a tiny radio frequency chip containing essential data in the form of an electronic product code will allow supply chain stakeholders to track the chain of custody, or as it is called, pedigree of every unit of medication on an individual basis.

Tremendous progress is being made in the development of technology. It is a monumental endeavor. It is going to require a lot of collaboration among all key players in the supply chain in order to get this technology instituted across our country. We are working closely with standard development organizations, for example, the EPC Global, to further the awareness and adoption of the EPC in health care both in the United States and abroad, and we have been an advocate for the adoption of this technology here in this country.

FDA's November 15, 2004, issuance compliance guide for implementing RFID feasibility study and pilot programs we think was an important and essential step in getting the technology off the ground. It will take an unwavering commitment from both the government and each of the supply chain partners to realize the adoption of this RFID technology in any kind of measured or meaningful way.

Finally, the entire supply chain and HDMA are constantly working to identify new ways and developing voluntary business practices that will assure product safety. In conclusion, we recognize the public trust placed upon them to ensure that our members provide authentic pharmaceutical products that are handled, stored and ultimately dispensed to patients safely and efficiently. Our message to the committee today is that securing the Nation's prescription drug supply requires a constant vigilance in the face of increasingly sophisticated international threats.

We do not believe there is a single solution to the effort; rather, a combination of approaches involving both government and supply chain partners. We think technology will play an important role, but technology is evolving and has to be combined with stricter regulations and best business practices. Any consideration of the importation of drugs from abroad must incorporate, we think, these multiple strategies. The health and safety of our Nation, literally, is at stake.

Thank you very much.

[The prepared statement of Mr. Gray follows:]

PREPARED STATEMENT OF JOHN M. GRAY

Thank you, Mr. Chairman and members of the committee for this opportunity to provide testimony on current efforts to further ensure and strengthen the integrity of the Nation's prescription drug supply. I appreciate the opportunity to provide the perspective of the domestic healthcare distribution industry as this committee considers the issue of importation of prescription drug products from abroad.

My name is John Gray, and I am the President and CEO of the Healthcare Distribution Management Association (HDMA). For more than 125 years, HDMA has worked with its members—the Nation's 46 full-service healthcare distributors—to secure a safe, efficient and reliable distribution system that provides life-saving healthcare products and services. On any given day, HDMA's member companies are responsible for delivering 9 million of the Nation's prescription drug products to more than 130,000 retail pharmacies, hospitals, nursing homes, clinics and other provider sites in all 50 States.

My purpose here today is to emphasize four principal points:

1. The primary responsibility of the healthcare industry is to ensure patient health and safety.

2. Our mission as healthcare distributors is to ensure that the prescription drug supply chain remains safe, secure and tightly regulated. Any efforts to permit the importation of prescription drug products from abroad must not weaken this system.

3. Significant efforts are underway, and must continue, to further secure the domestic supply chain in the face of increasing incidents of counterfeit and adulterated products entering markets, both domestic and abroad.

4. There is no single solution to secure the integrity of the prescription drug supply—the only effective response is one that involves multiple strategies and includes the participation and commitment of all supply chain partners.

Patients in the United States expect that when they receive a prescription from their medical provider, the medication will be available for dispensing upon their arrival at a pharmacy. They expect and deserve authentic medicine that has been handled and stored properly. Each member of the supply chain—from the manufacturer, to the distributor, to the pharmacy—has an important role and we must work in tandem to ensure a safe and reliable supply of prescription drugs for patients.

CURRENT REGULATORY ENVIRONMENT

The responsibility to provide a safe and reliable supply of prescription drugs requires constant vigilance. The Nation's drug distribution system is highly regulated at both the Federal and State levels of government, under the Prescription Drug Marketing Act[1] (PDMA), which was enacted in 1988 and amended in 1992. At the time of the PDMA's original enactment, Congress found that "American consumers [could not] purchase prescription drugs with the certainty that the products [were] safe and effective," and that there [was] an "unacceptable risk that counterfeit, adulterated, misbranded, subpotent, or expired drugs will be sold to American consumers."[2] The PDMA established a closed and highly regulated domestic supply chain. The PDMA also established minimum Federal licensing standards and delegated to the States the responsibility to serve as the licensing bodies. The States, therefore, are empowered to inspect, regulate and approve the firms conducting business as pharmaceutical distributors.

HDMA full service distributor members are also strictly regulated by the Drug Enforcement Administration (DEA), both as distributors of List I Chemicals and Controlled Substances. The DEA, along with State Controlled Substance Authorities, add an additional and important level of inspection and regulation of our member facilities, ensuring that products with abuse potential are kept in a highly secure environment with strong recordkeeping requirements.

This Federal/State regulatory and oversight partnership has served the Nation well to date. However, even the United States is not immune from the growing and increasingly sophisticated threat of counterfeiting. According to FDA's report entitled, "*Combating Counterfeit Drugs*" (February, 2004), patients in some countries actually have a better chance of getting a fake drug than the legitimate product. While still extremely rare, instances of counterfeit or adulterated[3] products entering the domestic supply chain have been on the increase in recent years. According to the FDA, the number of instances where counterfeit products have breached the domestic supply chain has increased from 6 cases in the year 2000 to 22 cases in 2003. Each of these situations poses a serious public health threat. As healthcare distributors, we recognize there is no greater responsibility than doing everything we can to ensure that the products we deliver to pharmacies and other healthcare providers are authentic, and have been stored and handled properly.

ONGOING SUPPLY CHAIN IMPROVEMENTS

Given the increasing sophistication and frequency of product counterfeiting, it is imperative that our Nation remains vigilant and constantly seeks new approaches

---

[1] Pub.L.No. 100–293 (1988) (codified as amended at 21 U.S.C. § 353 et seq. (1992)).

[2] *Id.* §§ 2(1), 2(8).

[3] A drug is deemed legally adulterated unless it is manufactured and held in conformance with current good manufacturing practice (GMP). GMP is intended, among other things, to assure that drugs are properly handled and stored at all times before they are dispensed to consumers. 21 U.S.C. § (a)(2)(D)

to further secure the domestic prescription drug supply. These ongoing efforts include:

1. strengthening government regulation, oversight and enforcement;
2. adopting new technologies; and
3. developing and implementing industry best practices.

1. STRENGTHENING GOVERNMENT REGULATION, OVERSIGHT & ENFORCEMENT

With regard to the strengthening of regulations that provide oversight and licensure of domestic healthcare distributors, HDMA joined in the FDA's call for States to review and revise their current wholesale licensing statutes and regulations. HDMA has taken the added step of drafting model legislation that is under consideration in multiple States. This HDMA model bill calls for additional requirements to be met in order to receive a prescription drug distribution license, as well as increased State oversight and enforcement measures.

While many States have taken their licensure and inspection responsibilities seriously, we remain concerned that too few States have devoted sufficient attention or resources to this area. For example, some States will issue a distribution license without ever conducting a pre-license inspection. Many States struggle with the ability to regulate out-of-state distributors in an industry that is increasingly shipping products across State lines. Many States also are slow to update and make publicly available the licensing status of a distributor or pharmacy.

HDMA believes that significant variation in the levels of State regulations of pharmaceutical distributors has led to inconsistent standards being applied across the States. We believe this must change and we will continue to advocate for stronger, more uniform national standards for the licensure of pharmaceutical distributors. HDMA believes an essential responsibility of government is to ensure that only legitimate, law-abiding organizations are licensed to distribute pharmaceutical products.

2. ADOPTING NEW TECHNOLOGIES

HDMA strongly believes that technology can serve an important role in securing the Nation's prescription drug supply; however, no single technology can absolutely prevent counterfeiting. Rather, a layering of various strategies can create a significant barrier to entry. Overt and covert authentication technologies currently are being used by manufacturers today.

As those who seek to introduce counterfeit or adulterated products into the supply chain become more sophisticated, so, too, must the technologies that manufacturers, distributors and pharmacies employ to frustrate and defeat them. We believe technologies employing electronic product codes (EPC)/radio frequency identification (RFID) hold the most promise for tracking, tracing and authenticating a product's movement across the supply chain. Using RFID technology, a tiny radio frequency chip containing essential data in the form of an electronic product code will allow supply chain stakeholders to track the chain of custody (or pedigree) of every unit of medication on an individual basis. By tying each discrete product unit to a unique electronic ID, a product can be tracked electronically through the supply chain.

Further, EPC/RFID technology represents an opportunity to significantly improve efficiencies in managing supplies and inventory. According to a recent HDMA Healthcare Foundation Report entitled, "*Adopting EPC in Healthcare: Costs and Benefits,*" patient safety can be enhanced and efficiencies to the healthcare supply chain can be achieved via the industry-wide adoption of EPC/RFID. EPC/RFID is more efficient and cost-effective than paper pedigrees or alternative electronic tracking methods that do not involve the serialization of individual products. Paper pedigrees have been forged in previous domestic counterfeiting situations. Moreover, paper pedigrees would literally halt the efficient distribution of drugs given the volume of products delivered and the sophisticated automation technology utilized to do so safely and efficiently.

I am pleased to report to the committee that tremendous progress is being made in the development and adoption of EPC/RFID technology with respect to pharmaceutical products. This is a monumental endeavor that will require close collaboration among all constituents of the healthcare supply chain and will take several years to proliferate the market in the United States. Industry, commercial vendors and government agencies are working together to develop the necessary standards for communication of tagged items across the supply chain. HDMA is working closely with standards development organizations such as EPCglobal to further the awareness, adoption and implementation of EPC in healthcare. While progress is extremely positive, there are many hurdles to overcome including business and technology challenges such as data management issues, interoperability of tags and readers and standards development. HDMA's focus has been to advocate for the adoption of this technology in the United States.

FDA's November 15, 2004 issuance of a Compliance Policy Guide (CPG) for implementing RFID feasibility studies and pilot programs was an important and essential step in moving this technology forward. The policy guide clarified the Agency's position with regard to any labeling or current Good Manufacturing Practices (GMP) issues that may arise by affixing an RFID tag to a pharmaceutical product. Several manufacturers and distributors simultaneously announced their intention to move forward with pilot programs that will involve the tagging of products susceptible to counterfeiting. These studies will significantly enhance the understanding and operability of this technology in the healthcare system.

Although the industry is moving forward in the development and adoption of EPC/RFID technology, it will take time and an unwavering commitment on the part of government and each partner in the supply chain to realize adoption of RFID technology in a measured, meaningful and universal way. HDMA members look forward to the support of the committee in ensuring that our laws and regulations continue to support the adoption of this important and patient safety enhancing technology.

3. DEVELOPING AND IMPLEMENTING INDUSTRY BEST PRACTICES

Finally, the entire supply chain is constantly identifying new ways to improve upon business practices that can enhance product safety. Many of HDMA's full service distributor members have adopted a voluntary set of best practices known as the "Recommended Guidelines for Pharmaceutical Distribution System Integrity." These guidelines establish a rigorous due diligence process for pharmaceutical distributors in order to further protect the integrity of the pharmaceutical supply chain.

CONCLUSION

In conclusion, HDMA members recognize the public trust placed upon them to ensure that authentic pharmaceutical products are handled, stored and ultimately, dispensed to patients safely and efficiently. Our message to the committee today is that securing the Nation's prescription drug supply chain requires constant vigilance in the face of increasingly sophisticated threats. We do not believe there is a single solution to this effort; rather, a combination of many approaches is required, involving the government and all supply chain partners. Technology plays an important and essential role in this effort, but technology is evolving and must be combined with strict regulation and best business practices to be most effective. Any consideration of the importation of prescription drugs from abroad must, at a minimum, incorporate these multiple approaches to safety and security. The health and safety of our Nation, literally, is at stake.

HDMA appreciates this opportunity to provide the perspective of the Nation's full-service healthcare distributors on these critically important issues.

The CHAIRMAN. Thank you.

Mr. Carmen Catizone.

STATEMENT OF CARMEN A. CATIZONE, MS, RPH, DPH, EXECUTIVE DIRECTOR/SECRETARY, NATIONAL ASSOCIATION OF BOARDS OF PHARMACY

Mr. CATIZONE. Thank you, Mr. Chairman, Senator Kennedy, other members of the committee. I am honored to be here today and respond to the committee's request on if and how the National Association of Boards of Pharmacy Verified Internet Pharmacy Practice Site Program could be utilized to help assure the safety of drugs purchased over the Internet if the United States were to legalize drug importation.

The VIPPS program was introduced in 1999 by NABP and incorporates traditional regulation and licensure with consumer empowerment to help consumers discern legal and legitimate pharmacies from rogue pharmacies. The VIPPS program allows consumers to make an educated choice about what pharmacies they should use and directs them to licensed and regulated pharmacies. There is no other program in the world that matches the VIPS program. The majority of programs representing themselves as accreditation or certification bodies for Internet pharmacies are simply promotional vehicles for Internet entrepreneurs and charlatans.

In NABP's opinion, the only means of providing assurances for the importation of medications into the United States is the development of a sound regulatory framework that allows only drug products that are approved by the FDA and manufactured in FDA-registered facilities to be imported in the United States for dispensing to U.S. patients through U.S.-licensed pharmacists and pharmacies. Clearly, the VIPPS program can be implemented to ensure that foreign pharmacies and wholesale distributors are dispensing medications in accordance with State and Federal laws.

To structure an importation model, NABP would define a new category within its VIPPS program: an international VIPPS patient care pharmacy that would identify VIPPS-accredited pharmacies outside the United States. NABP would amend the VIPPS criteria to address international practice and focus on areas that document and provide evidence on an ongoing basis that the drug products being distributed were FDA-approved and originated from FDA-registered facilities. This discussion would focus, again, on the pedigree, which has been mentioned several times in the hearing.

We would also work with United States and foreign pharmacy licensing authorities to develop mutual enforcement agreements with the pharmacy jurisdictions in the United States and other countries that would regulate international pharmacies by requiring the licensure, registration of these entities by the appropriate authority in the country where the facility is located as well as where the patient resides.

As importation has evolved, the model has changed. We have seen the medications go from the pharmacy to the patient, from the pharmacy to a wholesale distributor to the patient, from the wholesale distributor to the pharmacy to the patient. It is critical to include the entire process in the regulatory model so that the loop is closed, and the integrity of the U.S. distribution system is maintained.

On this important note, serious consideration should be given to the regulation and the accreditation of foreign wholesale distributors. NABP's Verified, Accredited Wholesale Distributors Program, which is now in operation and was created in response to the FDA's report on counterfeit drugs, provides a mechanism for the States and for the industry to accredit prescription drug and device distributors that helps to ensure the safety of the U.S. drug distribution system and thwart the introduction of counterfeit products.

In closing, NABP appreciates the opportunity to share our comments with the committee. We respectfully request that the committee recognize that allowing and encouraging the illegal purchase and importation of prescription medications from other countries without the appropriate regulatory safeguards is a serious threat to our regulatory foundation and patient safety. NABP requests further the committee's consideration and assistance in preserving the sanctity of current regulations, so as to prevent patients from being seriously injured by the illegal importation of drug products from countries where U.S. laws and regulations are being ignored or the laws and standards for drug safety and patient care are below the standards here in the United States

NABP also respectfully asks consideration to the importance of Federal and State laws, maintaining the FDA drug approval and monitoring process, and the adoption of solutions that are focused on patient safety such as the VIPPS and VAWDS programs. Thank you.

[The prepared statement of Mr. Catizone follows:]

PREPARED STATEMENT OF CARMEN A. CATIZONE

Chairman Enzi and members of the committee, I am honored to respond to the request of the committee and present information concerning the National Association of Boards of pharmacy (NABP) Verified Internet Pharmacy Practice Sites (VIPPS) program. Hopefully this information can/will assist the committee in determining if and how the VIPPS program could be utilized to help assure the safety of drugs purchased over the Internet if the United States were to legalize drug importation.

The NABP was founded in 1904. Our members are the pharmacy regulatory and licensing jurisdictions in the United States, District of Columbia, Guam, Puerto Rico, and the Virgin Islands, eight provinces of Canada, two Australian States, New Zealand, and South Africa. Our purpose is to serve as the independent, international, and impartial Association that assists States and provinces in developing, implementing, and enforcing uniform standards for the purpose of protecting the public health.

In May, 2004, we appeared before the Health and Human Services' (HHS) Task Force on Importation chaired by Richard H. Carmona, M.D., M.P.H., F.A.C.S., United States Surgeon General. At that time we stated NABP's opposition to the illegal importation of drug products and presented information to document the compromise of our medication system and State regulation of the practice of pharmacy that is occurring because of the illegal importation of drug products. Our testimony also noted that the member States of NABP adopted a resolution which resolved:

That NABP continue to oppose the illegal importation of medications and express to the Food and Drug Administration (FDA) the concerns of its member boards and strongly urge the FDA or appropriate legal authority to pursue actions against State and local governments for endorsing, promoting, or engaging in the illegal importation of medications.

The illegal importation of drugs from Canada and other countries is one of the most complicated and frustrating issues confronting pharmacy regulators. It is an issue that has the potential of altering how drugs are approved, medications are dispensed in the United States, and the practice of pharmacy is regulated. In fact, if the illegal importation of drugs into the United States is allowed to continue unabated, the impact on patient safety will be devastating. Patients illegally importing drugs are bypassing the drug approval process of the Food and Drug Administration (FDA) and the safety of U.S. licensed pharmacists and pharmacies and placing their health and well being in the hands of the country, territory, or back room with the seemingly, lowest prices for drugs.

Critics of the regulatory actions of the FDA and State boards of pharmacy against entities illegally distributing or assisting in the illegal distribution of drugs from countries outside of the United States contend that there have been only a few reports of patient harm and injury. Although the number of reports may be low, the actual harm to patients could be significant. NABP maintains that the number of reported patient injuries is low and immeasurable because patients may not be able to discern whether the drugs received from other countries are authentic or appropriate and adverse reactions resulting from patients receiving wrong or counterfeit drugs may not manifest in the health care system until sometime later when the patient's condition worsens and requires emergency treatment or hospitalization. NABP also maintains that consumers purchasing drugs from other countries are reluctant to report any adverse consequences because of the fear of prosecution that could result for violating Federal and State laws.

NABP'S VERIFIED INTERNET PHARMACY PRACTICE SITES™ (VIPPS®) PROGRAM

The Verified Internet Pharmacy Practice Sites Program (VIPPS) was introduced by NABP in 1999 and incorporates traditional regulation and consumer empowerment into a thorough and successful accreditation and certification system. The VIPPS program was implemented with wide consumer acceptance and support. Information about the VIPPS program has appeared on national and local news media programs and consumer information specials. The exposure included programming on CNN, ABC World News Tonight, NPR Radio, NBC News, CBS News, and Fox Special Report. Articles, stories and consumer advice recommending the VIPPS program have also appeared throughout the print media in local newspapers across the country as well as in Time, Newsweek, the Ladies Home Journal, Consumer Reports, USA Today, Wall Street Journal, New York Times, Washington Post, and other national publications. NABP estimates that more than 10 million consumers have heard, watched, or read about the VIPPS program. Government agencies such as the FDA and the Center for Medicare and Medicaid Services (CMS) also reference and recommend that consumers refer to the VIPPS program. Professional organizations such as the Federation of State Medical Boards (FSMB), American Pharmacists Association (APhA), and the American Medical Association (AMA) have also referenced and recommended consumers to the VIPPS program to consumers.

The VIPPS accreditation program is similar to the national accreditation of hospitals recognized by Federal and State agencies and health care insurance companies. The VIPPS program addresses the Internet pharmacy's level of performance in key functional areas and focuses on an Internet pharmacy's ability to provide safe medications and quality care. The VIPPS program is unique to the practice of pharmacy and the Internet. There are no equal or equivalent accreditation or certification programs in the world. Other certification or accreditation programs which operate in the Internet arena lack NABP's extensive evaluation process, access to licensure and disciplinary information, and intense onsite inspection procedures. The majority of programs representing themselves as accreditation or certification bodies for Internet pharmacies are simply promotional vehicles for Internet entrepreneurs and charlatans.

The VIPPS process ensures compliance with State and Federal laws governing the practice of pharmacy and verifies directly with the State boards of pharmacy the licensure and disciplinary status of the Internet pharmacy seeking accreditation. VIPPS also certifies compliance with an 18-point criterion (Attachment A) through rigorous onsite inspections and the meticulous analysis of the site's operations and submitted written information. The VIPPS Criteria include criterion that concentrate on the distinctions of Internet practice, such as the transmission of prescription information and patient data, confidentiality of patient records, and quality improvement and monitoring of prescription processing and patient interactions.

The VIPPS Criteria also set forth performance expectations for activities that affect the integrity of the medications and quality of patient care. If an Internet pharmacy does the right things and does them well, there is a strong likelihood that its patients will experience good outcomes. NABP develops its criteria in consultation with health care experts, providers, measurement experts, regulators, and consumers. Achieving VIPPS accreditation is an indication that the Internet pharmacy is recognized for complying with national performance standards that promote safe medications and quality healthcare delivery.

In early 2003, NABP detected a major shift in activity on the Internet. At this time, there appeared to be an unprecedented increase in the number of Internet Web sites offering American consumers lower priced medications from Canada and other foreign sources. Sites involved in this illegal activity jammed the Internet, deluged consumers with advertisements and solicitations at every turn and click, and aggressively lobbied senior citizen groups and other special interest groups for Congressional support to protect their activities. NABP spoke out at the time, and continues to speak out, against these sites and their illegal activities. NABP has commented extensively on the need to close these sites and end their illegal operations. Working with the States and the FDA, NABP has documented incidences of patient harm from Internet sites and pharmacies operating in Canada and other parts of the world. Most recently, with the proliferation of Canadian Internet pharmacies exporting prescription medications to the United States, NABP has discovered surreptitious Web sites designed to look like they are based in Canada, when in actuality they are operated in and/or ship medications from Latin America or overseas and have no ties to Canada other than their misappropriation of the Canadian flag.

In November of 2003, NABP and the National Association of Pharmacy Regulatory Authorities (NAPRA) in Canada expanded the VIPPS program to include legitimate, legal, and safe pharmacies duly registered in the various provinces. The

VIPPS Canada program mirrors NABP's VIPPS program in the United States and identifies for Canadian patients Internet pharmacies accredited through a credible process with standards focusing on the protection of the public health and patient safety. Presently, those Canadian pharmacies which ship prescription drugs into the United States, in direct violation of State and Federal laws, would not qualify for VIPPS certification.

VIPPS: WHETHER AND HOW THIS TYPE OF PROGRAM COULD HELP ASSURE THE SAFETY OF DRUGS PURCHASED OVER THE INTERNET IF THE UNITED STATES WERE TO LEGALIZE DRUG IMPORTATION

The importation of medications into the United States from Canadian and other non-U.S. based pharmacies poses a public health concern and regulatory quagmire. The public health concern rests with the inability of foreign and U.S. pharmacy regulators to ensure that medications illegally imported into the United States are legitimate and safe because the importation activities fall outside of the existing regulatory safeguards. The regulatory position advocated by NABP emphasizes the importance of ensuring that the dispensing and distribution of medications in the United States are safe for American patients.

The only means of providing such assurances is the development of a sound regulatory framework that allows *only* drug products that are approved by the FDA and manufactured in FDA registered facilities to be imported in the United States for dispensing to U.S. patients from U.S. licensed pharmacists and pharmacies. If the appropriate inter-border regulatory framework is not in place, then allowing for the purchase and import of drugs from pharmacies or foreign operations that do not comply with existing Federal and State laws and regulations places U.S. patients at significant risk. If the safeguards in place for the U.S. drug approval system and State regulation of pharmacists and pharmacies and wholesale distributors are not in place or deliberately compromised, then U.S. patients will be subject to the dangers of a "buyers beware" environment and left unprotected to gamble with their health and safety.

More importantly, each progression to extend the distribution source of drugs outside of the FDA drug approval process and U.S. licensed pharmacists and pharmacies to unknown borders exacerbates an already dangerous situation. The importation of drugs without an effective regulatory framework to countries lacking valid drug approval processes, regulatory systems, or practice standards, provides for the almost certain erosion and destruction of the entire drug approval process and regulatory structure of the United States. Allowing the illegal importation of drugs to continue will, in effect, turn back the hands of time to the days of the Elixir Sulfanilamide disaster (1937) when 105 people died after ingesting a preparation containing diethylene glycol, anti-freeze. It was a time before the FDA was charged to ensure the safety of drugs and the drug development strategy was to throw drugs together and if they didn't explode, they were appropriate to sell.

The U.S. system, based within the regulatory framework of State practice acts and the FDA drug approval and monitoring processes, has been exemplary in protecting the citizens of the various States and providing patients and health care practitioners with the assurances and confidence that the medications prescribed and dispensed are safe and effective products. The State-based regulatory system successfully protects patients and is flexible enough to extend the regulatory framework and safety net across State borders and allow for the practices of telepharmacy and telemedicine.

A discussion of whether the VIPPS Program or a VIPPS model can be utilized to allow for the importation of drugs is mute if the violation of Federal laws and compromise of the FDA drug approval process are not addressed and corrected. Clearly the VIPPS program can be implemented to ensure that foreign pharmacies and wholesale distributors are dispensing and distributing medications, respectively, in accordance with State and Federal laws. This can be accomplished through the following modifications of the VIPPS program:

(1) NABP would define an *International VIPPS Patient Care Pharmacy* agreement to certify VIPPS accredited pharmacies outside of the United States. NABP would amend the VIPPS Criteria to require pharmacies dispensing medications across the border and seeking VIPPS accreditation to document and provide evidence on an ongoing basis that the drug products being distributed were FDA approved and obtained from FDA registered facilities. The international pharmacy seeking VIPPS accreditation would also have to document and demonstrate compliance with the laws and the patient care standards of all jurisdictions in which the patient and the pharmacy resides.

(2) NABP would work with U.S. and foreign pharmacy authorities to develop mutual enforcement agreements with the pharmacy jurisdictions in other countries that would regulate international pharmacies by requiring the licensure/registration of these entities by the appropriate authority in the country where they are located and where the patient resides. The mutual enforcement agreements would also require continued monitoring of the distribution and dispensing of medications in order to ensure that the pharmacy maintains its compliance with all applicable laws/regulations. This requirement could also be managed through the International VIPPS Patient Care Pharmacy program.

However, and most importantly, absent action to resolve the violations of Federal law, no modification of the VIPPS program is possible to create a legal and effective regulatory framework for the importation of medications to U.S. patients. Legislation passed in Rhode Island requiring the Rhode Island Board of Pharmacy to license Canadian pharmacies despite the obvious and knowing violation of Federal laws is a perilous and illogical action. The Rhode Island legislation is in effect requiring the agency mandated to uphold the pharmacy laws of the State to license pharmacies willfully engaged in violation of Federal laws in complete defiance of the legislative mandate of the State board. It is inconceivable to place such a confounding burden on the State board of pharmacy or to implement an importation model that does not recognize the necessity of complying with Federal law. Similarly, to implement a VIPPS-like program for the importation of drugs in direct violation of Federal law would not be feasible and defy the entire enforcement and legal system of the United States.

VERIFIED-ACCREDITED WHOLESALE DISTRIBUTORS™ (VAWD™) PROGRAM

On a final but very important note, if an importation model is advanced, provided Federal law is not violated, then serious consideration must be given to the regulation and accreditation of foreign wholesale distributors. NABP's Verified-Accredited Wholesale Distributors (VAWD) program, created in response to the FDA's Report on Counterfeit Drugs, provides a mechanism for the accreditation of prescription drug and device distributors that helps to ensure the safety of the U.S. drug distribution system and thwart counterfeit products. Similar to the VIPPS program, the VAWD program requires licensure verification, policy and procedure evaluation, and an onsite inspection to ensure compliance with comprehensive drug distribution laws and standards addressing such important issues as background checks, facility security, pedigrees, authentications, quarantine of suspect product, and verification of product sellers and purchasers. The VAWD program represents an additional regulatory model that can be utilized to oversee the safe cross-border distribution of prescription medications to U.S. wholesale distributors and pharmacies.

CONCLUSIONS

NABP appreciates the opportunity to share its comments with the committee. NABP respectfully requests that the committee recognize that allowing and encouraging the illegal purchase and importation of medications from other countries without the appropriate regulatory safeguards is a serious threat to our regulatory foundation and patient safety. NABP requests further, the committee's assistance in preserving the sanctity of current regulations so as to prevent any patient from being seriously injured by the illegal importation of drug products from countries where U.S. laws and regulations are being ignored or the laws and standards for drug safety and effectiveness of that country or territory are not equivalent to U.S. laws and standards. NABP also respectfully requests that if importation of medications to U.S. patients is allowed then careful consideration be given to the importance of Federal and State laws, maintaining the FDA drug approval and monitoring process, and the adoption of solutions that are focused on patient safety.

Thank you for the opportunity to address this important issue.

ATTACHMENT A.—VERIFIED INTERNET PHARMACY PRACTICE SITES (VIPPS) CRITERIA

LICENSURE AND POLICY MAINTENANCE

Qualifying VIPPS Pharmacies (see definitions) must:

(1) Provide NABP with the information necessary to verify that the VIPPS pharmacy is licensed or registered in good standing to operate a pharmacy and/or engage in the practice of pharmacy with all applicable jurisdictions;

(2) Provide NABP with the information necessary to verify that all persons affiliated with the site, including those affiliated through contractual or other responsible

arrangements, that are engaging in the practice of pharmacy are appropriately licensed or registered and in good standing in all applicable jurisdictions;

(3) Maintain and enforce a comprehensive policy and procedure that documents how the pharmacy's policies and procedures are organized, authorized for implementation, revised, retired and archived; and

(4) Comply with all applicable statutes and regulations governing the practice of pharmacy where licensed or registered, and comply with the more stringent law or regulation as determined by conflicts of law rules. VIPPS pharmacies must maintain and enforce policies and procedures that address conflicts of law issues that may arise between individual States or between State and Federal laws and regulations. Said policies and procedures must assure compliance with applicable laws including generic substitution laws and regulations, and must prohibit unauthorized therapeutic substitution from occurring without necessary patient or prescriber authorization and outside of the conditions for participation in State or Federal programs such as Medicaid.

PRESCRIPTIONS

Qualifying VIPPS Pharmacies, in accordance with applicable State and Federal laws and regulations, must:

(5) Maintain and enforce policies and procedures that assure the integrity, legitimacy, and authenticity of the Prescription Drug Order and seek to prevent Prescription Drug Orders from being submitted, honored, and filled by multiple pharmacies. Maintain and enforce policies and procedures that assure that prescription medications are not prescribed or dispensed based upon telephonic, electronic, or online medical consultations without there being a pre-existing patient-prescriber relationship that has included an in-person physical examination.

PATIENT INFORMATION

Qualifying VIPPS Pharmacies, in accordance with applicable State and Federal laws and regulations, must:

(6) Maintain and enforce policies and procedures ensuring reasonable verification of the identity of the patient, prescriber, and, if appropriate, caregiver, in accordance with applicable State law;

(7) Obtain and maintain in a readily accessible format, patient medication profiles and other related data in a manner that facilitates consultation with the prescriber, when applicable, and counseling of the patient or caregiver;

(8) Conduct a prospective drug use review (DUR) prior to the dispensing of a medication or device in accordance with applicable State law; and

(9) Maintain and enforce policies and procedures to assure patient confidentiality and the protection of patient identity and patient-specific information from inappropriate or non-essential access, use, or distribution while such information is being transmitted via the Internet and while the pharmacy possesses such information. [The NABP Guidelines for the Confidentiality of Patient Health Care Information as It Relates to Patient Compliance and Patient Intervention Programs can serve as a useful resource for addressing the confidentiality and security of patient data.]

COMMUNICATION

Qualifying VIPPS Pharmacies, in accordance with applicable State and Federal laws and regulations and VIPPS program criteria must:

(10) Maintain and enforce policies and procedures requiring pharmacists to offer interactive, meaningful consultation to the patient or caregiver;

(11) Maintain and enforce policies and procedures establishing a mechanism for patients to report, and the VIPPS Pharmacy to take appropriate action regarding, suspected adverse drug reactions and errors;

(12) Maintain and enforce policies and procedures that provide a mechanism to contact the patient and, if necessary, the prescriber, if an undue delay is encountered in delivering the prescribed drug or device. Undue delay is defined as an extension of the normal delivery cycle sufficient to jeopardize or alter the patient treatment plan;

(13) Maintain and enforce policies and procedures establishing mechanisms to inform patients or caregivers about drug recalls; and

(14) Maintain and enforce policies and procedures establishing mechanisms to educate patients and caregivers about the appropriate means to dispose of expired, damaged, and unusable medications.

STORAGE AND SHIPMENT

Qualifying VIPPS Pharmacies, in accordance with applicable State and Federal laws and regulations and VIPPS program criteria, must:

(15) Ship controlled substances to patients via a secure and traceable means; and

(16) Assure that medications and devices are maintained within appropriate temperature, light, and humidity standards, as established by the United States Pharmacopeia (USP), during storage and shipment.

OVER-THE-COUNTER PRODUCTS

Qualifying VIPPS Pharmacies must:

(17) Comply with all applicable Federal and State laws regarding the sale of Over-the-Counter Products identified as precursors to the manufacture or compounding of illegal drugs.

QUALITY IMPROVEMENT PROGRAMS

Qualifying VIPPS Pharmacies must:

(18) Maintain a Quality Assurance/Quality Improvement Program.

REPORTING TO NABP

Qualifying VIPPS Pharmacies must:

(19) Notify NABP within thirty (30) days of any change of information provided as part of the verification process, including change in pharmacist-in-charge, or involving data displayed on the VIPPS Web site. VIPPS pharmacies shall notify NABP in writing within ten (10) days of ceasing operations. The written notification shall include the date the pharmacy will be closed, and an affirmation that all VIPPS Seals and references to the VIPPS program have been removed from the Web site and wherever else they are displayed.

The CHAIRMAN. Thank you very much.

Dr. Peter Rost.

STATEMENT OF PETER ROST, M.D., VICE PRESIDENT OF MARKETING FOR ENDOCRINE CARE, PFIZER

Dr. ROST. Thank you, Chairman Enzi, Senator Kennedy. Thank you so much for inviting me here today.

My name is Peter Rost, and I am a physician who has spent 20 years marketing pharmaceuticals. I have been responsible for a region in Europe, and I am currently a vice-president with Pfizer. The views I will present today are my own and do not reflect those of my employer, which will become abundantly clear.

By now, most of you have noticed that I do not have an East Coast accent. I am a naturalized U.S. citizen, came to this country, voted with my feet, because I wanted to be here. I think this is a wonderful country, a country where we have freedom of speech, a freedom that I am choosing to exercise today.

The first question I usually get is you are a drug executive. How can you speak in favor of reimportation? That does not make any sense. What has influenced me is my own personal experience with reimportation in Europe, working for another pharmaceutical company. I first assisted the President of Europe, and then, I was managing the northern region in Europe, and I had a problem over there, I had a problem of a lot of reimported drugs coming into my market, and I was not happy. So you know what I did? I lowered my prices 30 to 40 percent. Do you know what happened? In 2 years, I doubled sales. My market company went from number 19 in the business to number 7, less than 2 years, best performance in the history of the Swedish pharmaceutical industry.

So I learned that the free market works and that there are several sides to this coin, and I think that the industry is making a historic mistake right now opposing drug importation, and I am not the only one thinking so. As a matter of fact, Roy Vagelos, the well-known former chairman of Merck and one of the industry's most prominent boosters last year in the New York Times said the industry delivered miracles, and now, they are throwing it all away. They just do not get it. He was referring to drug prices.

I am going to focus on two areas: safety and cost-effectiveness of reimportation. Lester Crawford has been quoted as saying that his main concern about reimportation is that Al Qaeda would attack the supply of drugs. But being concerned about safety of imported drugs assumes that you are safe already. I do not think we are. What the FDA has forgotten is that we have thousands of secondary wholesalers in the United States today. States license them, not the FDA. All it takes for a terrorist to become a drug wholesaler is $1,000 and a driver's license.

Another problem, very important, right here in the United States today is that our drugs are shipped in big vats to wholesalers, and they pour them in smaller bulk-size bottles, and then, the pharmacists pour those drugs to the patients, lots of entry points for a terrorist or anyone else. In Europe, it is different. Drugs are shipped in individual bottles or blisters, and no one touches the drug after it leaves the manufacturer. Pretty good system. We should have it, too.

So I believe that getting drugs from Europe really could be safer than getting it in the United States. The German Federal Health Ministry has recently verified that not one single confirmed case of a counterfeit medicine has ever come through the trade chain in Europe.

Legalized and regulated reimportation is about the safe drug supply. It is about getting drugs to consumers who cannot afford them, because, you know, the biggest safety problem we have, the safety problem nobody has mentioned today is when you do not take a drug. It does not work. We have lots of patients in the United States that do not take drugs: 15 percent of uninsured children did not take the drugs they needed because of cost. Twenty-eight percent of adults, same thing. Diabetes care had a study showing that 28 percent of elderly diabetes patients had to choose between food and drugs in America today.

What is the effect of this? We have the numbers. I just checked out the WHO Web site. In America, more babies die every year than any other industrialized country and more elderly die. We have higher infant mortality rates, child mortality rates and a shorter life span than every other industrialized country: Singapore, Australia, New Zealand, Japan, Canada, Western Europe.

Now, I remember this was the country that put a man on the moon, and here we are 40 years later not even taking care of our babies. I mean, come on: this, we have to do something about. Drugs help people. Drugs make a difference. We know that. That is part of the solution.

You have also heard in the HHS report that savings would really only represent 1 to 2 percent of drug expenditures, and the biggest fallacy in the report is that it assumes that there would only be a 20 percent discount, while we know that drugs are 100 percent more expensive than in Europe. So this assumes that reimporters would really do price gouging.

I need to wrap up, so I will say that my overall concern is that every day, Americans die because they cannot afford life-saving drugs, because we want to protect the profits of often foreign corporations. I believe we have to speak out for the people who cannot afford drugs in favor of free trade and against the closed market. Stopping good reimportation bills has a high cost, not just in money but in American lives.

I and many of my colleagues joined the drug industry to save lives, not to take them. That is the reason I am here today. Thank you.

[The prepared statement of Dr. Rost follows:]

PREPARED STATEMENT OF PETER ROST

Chairman Enzi and Senator Kennedy thank you for inviting me today.

My name is Peter Rost and I'm a physician who has spent 20 years marketing pharmaceuticals. I've been responsible for a region in Europe and I'm currently a Vice President at Pfizer. The views I will present are my own and do not reflect those of my employer.

By now, most of you have noted that I don't have an East Coast accent. I'm a naturalized U.S. citizen and I voted with my feet when I came here 20 years ago. I think this is a great country, where we have the freedom of speech—a freedom I'm exercising today.

The first question I usually get is "you're a drug executive, how can you speak in favor of reimportation." What has influenced me is my own personal experience with reimportation in Europe while working for another pharmaceutical company. First I assisted the president of Europe; then I headed up the Nordic region. I had lots of reimported drugs coming into my market, and I was not happy about this. So I dropped my own prices. You know what happened? I doubled sales and increased my company ranking from No. 19 to No. 7 in less than 2 years. So I know that the free market works and I think the industry is making a historic mistake, opposing drug importation.

My concern is that we have 67 million Americans without insurance for drugs. Many of them don't get the drugs they need because they can't afford them, because drugs cost twice as much in the United States as in other countries.

And what really troubles me is that when we in the drug industry charge these high prices to the uninsured, we sell the rest of our drugs, right here in the United States, today, at the same low prices we charge in Canada and Europe. It's done through rebates. These are given to those with enough power to negotiate drug prices, such as the Department of Veterans Affairs and various pharmacy benefit mangers.

So the fight against reimportation is a fight to continue to charge our uninsured, our elderly, our poor, our weakest, full price, while giving everyone else a rebate. This is fundamentally unethical. This is not how we're supposed to treat our grandparents who built this country.

Legalized reimportation can help these people. The biggest argument against reimportation is safety. [According to AP, FDA Commissioner] Lester Crawford has said that his main concern about drug reimportation is that al Qaeda might attack the supply of Canadian drugs.

But the FDA has forgotten that we have thousands of secondary wholesalers that trade drugs. States license them, not the FDA. All it takes for a terrorist to become a drug wholesaler is $1,000 and a driver's license, [according to Aaron Graham, head of security for Purdue Pharma, quoted in the Providence Journal]. Another problem, right here in the United States, is that our drugs are shipped in big vats to wholesalers, and then poured into smaller, bulk-size containers, from which tablets are dispensed manually to the patient. Lots of entry points for a terrorist. In Europe, drugs are sold in tamper-proof individual bottles or blisters, and no one touches a drug after it leaves the manufacturer.

So I believe that getting a drug from Europe is actually safer than getting it in the United States. The German Federal Health Ministry has verified that not one single confirmed case of a counterfeit medicine has ever come through the parallel trade chain. The UK regulatory authority has described the level of pharmaceutical counterfeiting as "virtually undetectable" [according to European Association of Euro-Pharmaceutical Companies].

Legalized and regulated reimportation is about a safe drug supply. It's about getting drugs to consumers who can't afford them. The biggest problem we have today is that drugs don't work if you don't take them. The Kaiser Family Foundation reported [in a 2001 study] that 15 percent of uninsured children and 28 percent of uninsured adults had gone without prescription medication because of cost. The journal Diabetes Care recently reported [February, 2004] on a study of older adults with diabetes. Twenty-eight percent said they went without food to pay for drugs. Is this how we want to treat our elderly, force them to choose between food and medicines?

And by the way, not even the drug companies want to pay for brand name drugs anymore. Novartis, one of the largest foreign drug makers, was so concerned about drug costs that the CEO sent a memo to all U.S. employees urging them to choose more generics. He didn't realize the memo would make front page news [NJ Star-Ledger, Oct 15, 2004].

[Let's also point out that half of the largest pharmaceutical companies are foreign corporations [Novartis, Glaxo, Astra-Zeneca, Roche and Sanofi-Aventis]. Why should we allow foreigners to come in and gouge American tax payers? Perhaps we shouldn't allow them to charge us more than their own governments are prepared to pay for our drugs? In Europe that's called reference pricing.]

So what do these foreign companies do? They take out big ads in American newspapers [Glaxo] and tell us that reimportation is not safe, while they know full well that it's been done safely and cost-effectively in their own home markets, in Europe, for over 20 years.

And I know that some of you may tell me that reimportation is not the answer; the HHS report speculates that savings would represent only 1 percent to 2 percent of drug expenditures.

You know what, the short answer is that if this was true, reimportation of drugs would never have existed in Europe with much smaller price differentials than the United States, and it would never take off in the United States. Why, then, do you think, the drug industry spends so much time and money fighting reimportation? The answer is that the data in the HHS report don't support this conclusion.

There is one simple flawed assumption in the report that drives their incorrect conclusion. It's that "U.S. drug buyers may get discounts of only 20 percent or less, with the rest of the difference between U.S. and foreign prices going to commercial importers." This assumption is based on a London School of Economics study. Guess who sponsored that study? You got it—the drug industry [Johnson & Johnson, according to Pharma Marketing].

[In fact, table 7.2 in the HHS report shows that U.S. drug prices are 100 percent higher than in Europe. So the premise of less than 20 percent savings assumes price gouging by importers and a complete lack of competition. Of course, we in the industry know that is not how the free market works.]

Every day Americans die because they can't afford life-saving drugs, because we want to protect the profits of foreign corporations. I believe we have to speak out for the people who can't afford drugs, in favor of free trade and against a closed market. Stopping good reimportation bills has a high cost. Not just in money, but in American lives.

I and many of my colleagues joined the drug industry to save lives, not to take them. That's the reason I've chosen to speak out today. Thank you.

The CHAIRMAN. Thank you. I appreciate the testimony of all of the members of the panel. I particularly appreciate the work that you put into an even fuller testimony, which will, of course, be a part of the record, and I encourage everybody to take a look at that. I appreciate your doing the summary so that we can get to questions.

Governor Pawlenty, I want to congratulate you on your RxConnect, a very innovative and obviously very effective system, and I have a bunch of questions on the cost of that so that we can relate it to what our costs might be on a Federal level were we to do something similar, but that is a lot more detailed. I found that that kind of puts people to sleep. So I will stick with some things that might be of greater interest.

In a poll that was released last fall that supports importation beyond Canada, there was about a 30 to 40 percent approval of that. Do the Internet pharmacies that MinnesotaRxConnect has a relationship with in Canada get their medications from countries other than Canada, and do you extend the Web site approvals beyond Canada, and if so, is that disclosed to the consumers?

Governor PAWLENTY. Mr. Chairman, thank you for the question. To clarify, the pharmacies that we have identified in Canada are actual pharmacies. Just to be clear on the term Internet pharmacy, sometimes, that leads people to think there is a virtual operation; there is not a physical operation. These orders are placed, in most instances, via a fax order form that is downloaded from our Web site and then faxed to the pharmacy, so we do not even actually—the consumers do not even place the order over the Internet. They are placed on a fax that goes to the physical pharmacy.

In terms of the source of the drugs from Canadian pharmacies, it varies, but as a general expectation, we expect the drugs to be sourced from Canada or the United States. We are aware that in certain instances, they are sourcing the drugs from certain European countries as well.

The CHAIRMAN. Thank you.

Mr. Gray, even in a closed distribution system like we have in the United States, from time to time, counterfeit medicines have been able to enter our system. How do you answer critics who argue that if counterfeit drugs are already entering our closed system, what is the harm in expanding the marketplace internationally?

Mr. GRAY. Well, products have entered the system, and our obligation is to tighten that regulatory requirement on the points at which those products have entered the system, and we have been arguing for stiffer State licensing, more national uniform licensing standards to close those loopholes, and our responsibility and our objective here today is as distributors, as folks who look strictly at the supply chain, the logistics aspects of the business, our feeling and our responsibility, we feel, is to make as secure our U.S. domestic supply chain before we start introducing foreign products into our system.

We acknowledge there are improvements to be made; there are stricter regulations, more uniform regulations that are required. There are technologies that need to be employed, and we think looking at the 50-State supply chain we currently handle, we have got enough to do there to make that supply chain as safe and secure and then start considering what other options there might be.

The CHAIRMAN. Thank you.

Mr. Catizone, I have heard arguments that the pharmacies in Canada or other developed countries are about the same as the pharmacies in the United States. Is that true, and if not, what are the differences that would be important for us to recognize?

Mr. CATIZONE. We have heard that same statement, Senator, and the fact of the matter is that the Canadian pharmacies that are licensed under the Canadian system are equivalent to the U.S. pharmacies and regulatory system. We cannot make that same statement for countries outside of Canada, because we have done an analysis of their practice standards, we have done an analysis of their products, and it appears that those standards and those product standards are below the standards within the United States.

The problem with importation is that it falls outside of the traditional regulatory schemes of Canada and the United States, and many pharmacies are operating within that empty wasteland and practicing and sending medicines to U.S. citizens without any regulation.

The CHAIRMAN. I will try and get some more information on that from you.

Mr. Rost, instead of us worrying about the reimportation thing, why do you not just reduce the price of the drugs in this country that you control, and then, we would not have to bring them back in through Canada?

Dr. ROST. Well, companies already do that. Companies today sell their drugs, which is not very much talked about, at European and Canadian prices today in the United States. They sell them to the parties who can negotiate: pharmacy benefit managers, Department of Veterans Affairs. The people who pay full price are the people who cannot negotiate: the uninsured, the poor, the elderly. They are the ones who get stuck with the high bill. I believe that is unethical.

The CHAIRMAN. Thank you. My time is expired. I do have some other questions for all of you. I will submit those in writing.

Senator KENNEDY. Dr. Rost, do you still work for Pfizer?

Dr. ROST. Yes, I do. Yes, I do.

Senator KENNEDY. Are they an enlightened company to let you loose up here?

[Laughter.]

Dr. ROST. Well, Pfizer reacted quite strongly the first time I was down here on the Hill, and they hired a law firm and started I would call it a bit of an inquisition, McCarthy-type hearing. They asked me about everything Senators and Congressmen had told me in their private chambers. They even asked me where I had slept when I was in Washington, and if anybody wonders, it was next to my wife.

[Laughter.]

But the Justice Department in New Jersey picked up on this and called me in, and it turns out that to try to dissuade anybody from appearing before Congress is a criminal act. You can get a year in jail. There are also State laws that protect people's legal political activity in their free time, which this is.

So after, I think, everybody was informed what the ground rules were, the investigation stopped.

Senator KENNEDY. Well, I was about to give them great credit for encouraging this kind of discourse from a person who is clearly a talented and concerned and experienced medical officer, but in any event, we are very grateful for your presence here and your testimony.

Governor, I just listened to one of the most persuasive Republicans I have ever heard with your very excellent commentary. You appeared before the task force. I am just wondering, it does not seem like the task force embraced your story. Just quickly, do you have any reactions to the task force or the task force report?

Governor PAWLENTY. Senator, I did appear before the task force and provided testimony. In listening to the Surgeon General, I think they viewed our approach or looking at it more critically beyond the scope of their charge from Congress. I will say the Surgeon General appeared to me and continues to appear to me to be genuine and sincere in his review of these matters. I would hope, though, that somebody would take a critical look at what Minnesota or other States are doing.

Senator KENNEDY. Okay.

Governor PAWLENTY. We have offered, by the way, to the FDA to be a demonstration project that we would pay for, have their inspectors come in. We would follow their rules. If there were problems, we would agree to shut down our program. They have not taken us up on the offer.

Senator KENNEDY. Well, it is an enormously impressive story.

Some of the pharmaceutical manufacturers are limiting the supplies of drugs to companies exporting drugs to Americans. Have your Canadian pharmacies been able to maintain adequate supplies for the Minnesotans?

Governor PAWLENTY. Senator, yes, but they are under increasing pressure, and more recently, we have signals that certain of the pharmacies are going to be running short or having delays or maybe running out of supply, because it is pretty clear that the pharmaceutical companies are choking off supply to those pharmacies because of their participation in our program.

Senator KENNEDY. The Surgeon General also commented, Governor, that it costs billions of dollars to inspect all of the drugs being shipped to individuals in the United States; do you feel it is necessary to inspect all of the packaged drugs that are sent from registered exporters to American consumers through the Federal Postal Service?

Governor PAWLENTY. Senator, no, I think the point that you raised earlier which is, again, the shiny object of—we concede, we stipulate that there are all sorts of garbage and shady characters on the Internet. We should not condone or promote that type of approach. What we should condone and promote is identifying and contractually engaging in a relationship and hopefully regulating established credible, reputable pharmacies, direct our consumers to those, and then, it just becomes a matter of shipping logistics, which I believe in an era, as we said, we put a man on the moon some years ago, we should at least be able to mail a package from Thunder Bay to Duluth without too much difficulty.

Senator KENNEDY. Dr. Rost, just if you would expand on this concept as a physician as well as a pharmaceutical company executive, is drug importation under a closely regulated environment a better alternative for consumers than not having access to the medicines because they cannot afford them?

Dr. ROST. Well, in Europe, they have a system up and running which they have had for over 20 years that works safely and cost-effectively which does not mean that consumers have to go on the Internet. This, what we have here today, is the Wild West. It is not good. I do not think anybody thinks it is good. What I am in favor of is the same thing as the American Medical Association is endorsing, which is a closed system, where wholesalers and pharmacists are up front importing drugs.

However, I know that takes time, and I believe when you see this boat, this sinking boat with babies and elderly, you cannot just sit around year after year after year and check on safety issues. If you have shown in a number of States and cities like Springfield, MA, that these programs work, let us get them running, because it can make a difference in the lives of a number of people.

We cannot wait. Every day we wait, we lose another person.

Senator KENNEDY. Thank you, Mr. Chairman. My time is up, I think.

The CHAIRMAN. Thank you.

Senator Alexander.

Senator ALEXANDER. Thank you, Mr. Chairman.

I wonder if any of you would help me evaluate the news report citing the Canadian Health Minister as suggesting that Canada does not want to be the drug store for the United States. What did you make of that? Was that an accurate statement? What does that mean?

Mr. CATIZONE. From our review of the situation, what it means, and our discussions with Canadian officials is one of the issues that was noted earlier: first, there is concern that there will not be medications for Canadian citizens because of the drain on the supply by U.S. patients, and second, the Canadian Government is also concerned that the medications and distributors dispensing those medications is falling outside of their regulated system, and they have no way to manage that or to respond to complaints that they are receiving from U.S. patients.

Senator ALEXANDER. Does anyone else have a comment on that?

Mr. GRAY. I would agree with that, and I think it is over the supply issue, because I know our companies have looked at this and are concerned about the issue given, as suggested earlier, 40 million people in Canada, 300 million people here, in the logistic supply chain sense, you look at it and say where do you get the volume of drugs to take care of 300 million Americans, most of who are fast approaching the age of 60 or over when you are only getting a small supply from Canada?

The question is when that drug comes over, and there is a limited supply, who makes the allocation decision as to where that drug goes? Does it go to Duluth, MN? Does it go to Phoenix, AZ? From our perspective we have looked at, we are trying to figure out where is all this drug supply going to come from to replace the drugs that we are currently selling in the United States at arguably or what is suggested to be maybe a cheaper price.

From a logistics point of view, we are questioning how we are going to get the drugs and how there are going to be enough of them.

Senator ALEXANDER. Dr. Rost.

Dr. ROST. Well, I think the sad situation we have today is that a number of large drug companies are limiting supply to Canada in the name of safety, but what really happens, then, is that they force Americans who cannot afford our drug prices in our drug stores here to buy those drugs somewhere else, which certainly does not help safety. The other comment I would have is clearly,

Canada cannot supply the United States. However, the European Union is a big market, and any functioning bill needs to include the European Union. To start with Canada would not work.

Senator ALEXANDER. Governor, did you have any reaction to that?

Governor PAWLENTY. Yes, Senator, just to put it in context, of course, people who are currently insured or are part of a program that has a prescription drug benefit are not the ones seeking Canada, so it is not the entire American market. It is just a slice of it. I think it is a supply issue as I understand the Canadian officials' concerns. That concern is really a function of the pharmaceutical companies limiting supply to Canada. It is not as if purchases that would have otherwise taken place in the United States, now that demand is transferred to Canada.

Theoretically, the supply could also then be diverted to Canada as more demand is generated in Canada, but what is happening, of course, is that the supply is being manipulated as a message, I think, to the Canadian pharmacies that you should not participate in these programs.

Senator ALEXANDER. Thank you. How can we most fairly evaluate what the costs would be of a system that would properly regulate and try to make safe imported drugs? I assume there would be—there has been some testimony about anticounterfeiting technology which might be developed, but I assume there would be an expense to that. Whenever the FDA testifies here on this subject, they talk to us about a fairly large cost of setting up the facilities to handle the importation of drugs. How do we evaluate whether taking this step would, in effect, with the added cost of anticounterfeiting technologies and other administrative costs, whether we would end up adding so much to the cost of the drugs that there really would not be much cost savings?

Mr. GRAY. Well, I think the first thing to consider, and the industry is in the process of doing this now, is what is the cost of this technology just within the domestic supply chain? We are actively working on pilot projects now with a number of organizations throughout the United States and in the industry already trying to understand what it is going to cost to implement just this system for track and trace within the 50 States.

I think until we have a grasp around that number, because that track and trace is going not only into pharmaceutical but consumer goods. Food industry and what have you are all quickly moving to it, and quite frankly, the suppliers of the technology and the implementers, those of us who are distributors, are trying to figure out what is this really going to cost, both the manufacturer cost, the distributor cost, the retail cost, the warehouse to operations cost and what have you.

Quite frankly, and as I said earlier, we have got to get our hands around the U.S. system first before we get an understanding what is going to be the implications of then extending this out beyond the U.S. borders, whether it is to Canada or the European Union. My adage is I think we have got to get our own house in order before we move outside to look at other systems. We have a lot of work still to do to get this technology into place for the next 3 to 4 years.

Senator ALEXANDER. Thank you.

I see my time is up. Thank you, Mr. Chairman.

The CHAIRMAN. Senator Burr.

Senator BURR. Thank you, Mr. Chairman, and I appreciate the fact that we are going to cover this issue over a number of hearings. I want to thank the witnesses and suggest this is probably one of the most important things this committee will do.

Governor, thank you for your willingness to come in. I think it is safe to say that what you exercise in Minnesota is, in fact, the waiver that the FDA provides individuals to seek the fulfillment of their prescriptions outside of the United States, something that they are not breaking the law to do today and that is not being enforced under any other method. The only change is that Canadians are now questioning whether the Canadian doctor's sign-off of a U.S. doctor's prescription should be policy; in other words, accepting the medical decisions of somebody in another country which, in fact, is what we are here discussing. Whether we are going to accept the medical decisions of the policies of other countries, and, as you said, I am comfortable in doing it with Canada, and I think as others have raised, if you cannot 100 percent with reliability understand the chain of custody—did that come from Italy. We could not sign onto any kind of harmonization agreement in the international community, because we disagree with many of the things that they use for their drug approval process.

We have a much bigger animal here that is not as simple as just trying to replicate what Minnesota has done. We have to look down the road and say how could it grow into something that was not intended on your part and certainly not intended on our part? I think you said that delivery was nothing to worry about. If delivery were nothing to worry about, part of the jurisdiction of this committee would not be bioterrorism. I would not be a subcommittee chairman concerned with the mail contamination of anthrax and ricin.

In fact, delivery is a concern. It is a concern in terrorism; it is a concern with adulterated products. It is a concern as to who we use, here in the United States, to verify whether it is an approved pharmacy or an approved outlet. Whether it is the Postal Service, whether it is Customs, and one only has to travel to Dulles Airport to see the challenge that a Customs agent has trying to determine whether a counterfeit drug which people have matched the identical color, the identical stamp, the identical packaging. I think Dr. Rost can agree to this, counterfeiting is rampant maybe not in our borders but around the country or around the world today.

I take for granted the shiny object was the question of safety, so I am not going to go to safety. But I think there are legitimate reasons that in an honest way, we can have that debate.

I want to go to U.S. Code. U.S. Code protects the patents of U.S. companies. The U.S. patent law protects the patents of U.S. companies. The Food, Drug and Cosmetic Act protects the patents of companies and products that are regulated by that agency. The Prescription Drug Marketing Act protects the patents of companies that are regulated under that marketing act.

Are you suggesting that we ignore U.S. Code, U.S. patent protection to facilitate a much broader access by U.S. consumers to prescription drugs?

Governor PAWLENTY. Senator, I hope my microphone is on. Senator, the question that you ask, I think, relates to intellectual property rights, and there are some who object to Canada's approach to either negotiating prices or how they deal with intellectual property. They do it somewhat differently than the United States does, but they have a framework for it, and it is public, and it is, you know, appropriate as far as they are concerned.

The concern that I have is when the United States is in the market for any other product, we shop the world for the best deal, and so, we go to China, for example, for products, even though they have a Communist Government, they have limited land rights, limited human rights, environmental policies that may be of concern to Americans. We do not get——

Senator BURR. But, Governor, let me stop you there. We aggressively go after textile products that come from China that are not authorized by the copyright holder. If, in fact, we have counterfeit CDs and DVDs, we are aggressively at the table negotiating with the Chinese today about the special nature of the way the United States protects those patents and those copyrights of U.S. innovators.

I guess my question is what do we do to the negotiators we have got at the table who are trying to negotiate the breakthroughs for 3M? 3M in your State has a tremendous list of patents. I think Dr. Rost would also agree that the ability to have patents allows innovation in the drug industry. I will come to you in a second.

I think that Senator Murray would agree that one of the reasons that Microsoft is headquartered in the United States is that we have a law that says we will protect your intellectual property. Yet we are picking one sector out now, and we are saying we are going to ignore that. The question is what precedent does this institution set if we ignore U.S. Code? This is rooted in the Constitution, and we are going to step on it.

Governor PAWLENTY. Senator, I do not understand that the Canadian patent system is somehow rogue or illegal or inappropriate. They have modern and sophisticated intellectual practices and property code in Canada.

Senator BURR. It is our patent system that I am—our patent system says that if it is against the patent holder's wishes, that product cannot be reimported or exported or imported into the United States. The question is are we going to enforce our own law, our own protections?

Governor PAWLENTY. Senator, I know time is short, but the system is, of course, that Canada negotiates with the pharmaceutical companies for their prices. They also negotiate over their patent protocols and procedures and expectations. It is a mutually negotiated or agreed-upon arrangement in Canada.

Senator BURR. But one thing is that reimportation into the United States is against U.S. Code, U.S. law. A patent holder would have to sign off on the reimportation, which is not the case when we move to a bulk situation.

Governor PAWLENTY. Senator, I understand your point. Now, as applied to the way that Minnesota does it, we fall within the individual use exception.

Senator BURR. Right.

Governor PAWLENTY. If Congress were to move more broadly into allowing this, then, you would have to address this issue. So I understand what you are saying now. It is not that it could not be done, but you would have to address it in a way that is fair and equitable.

Senator BURR. We would have to ignore U.S. law.

Governor PAWLENTY. If I might just quickly——

The CHAIRMAN. The Senator's time has expired. I will have to ask for each of you to respond to that in writing at this point——

Governor PAWLENTY. Okay.

The CHAIRMAN [continuing]. To any questions that he or the rest of us might have the same way, because the record will be left open for 10 days for witnesses to amplify their remarks and also members to propose different questions. I do thank the panel for the extensive knowledge that they have and their willingness to share it and to take the extra time to answer our written questions.

I would also ask unanimous consent that we be allowed to include a letter from Pfizer for the record to explain that Dr. Rost is not appearing on behalf of Pfizer.

Without objection.

[The information follows:]

PFIZER INC., CORPORATE AFFAIRS,
NEW YORK, NY,
February 16, 2005.

Hon. MICHAEL B. ENZI,
Chairman,
Committee on Health, Education, Labor, and Pensions,
Dirksen Senate Office Building,
Washington, D.C. 20510.

DEAR CHAIRMAN ENZI: We understand that Dr. Peter Rost will testify today before the Senate Committee on Health, Education, Labor, and Pensions on the subject of prescription drug importation. At the outset, it is important to note that while any citizen is entitled to speak before the Congress, Dr. Rost is not speaking on behalf of Pfizer. Dr. Rost has never been involved in the extensive analysis of this critical issue that has been undertaken at Pfizer. He has not participated in Pfizer's active involvement in the government's examination of this issue. These Pfizer activities include the following:

• In April, Pfizer's Vice President of Global Security, John Theriault, testified before the Department of Health and Human Services' Importation Task Force, which was mandated by Congress to study the feasibility of importation. In May, Pfizer provided a submission to the Task Force that supports Pfizer's position that foreign authorities do not have the controls in place to guarantee the safety of exported regulated drugs.

• Pfizer also participated in the GAO's study of drugs purchased online by helping determine whether these drugs are counterfeit. The GAO testified before a Senate subcommittee in June, concluding that consumers can easily buy drugs over the Internet without a prescription. The GAO concluded by stating, "It is notable that we identified these numerous problems despite the relatively small number of drugs we purchased, consistent with problems recently identified by State and Federal regulatory agencies."

In addition, we have no basis to support Dr. Rost's purported expertise in this area. It has been a number of years since Dr. Rost was stationed in Europe and we believe that his knowledge is outdated. For example, he incorrectly suggests that the price differences exploited by parallel trade in Europe have been passed on as savings to consumers when virtually all objective analysis refutes that assertion. A study conducted by the London School of Economics, which was published last year, found that national health systems within the EU realized minimal savings from parallel traded products. In fact, the study showed that no single national payer saved more than 2.2 percent because of this trade despite wildly varying price discrepancies. In the UK, the study found that "The impact on patients in the UK from parallel trade is zero" and that prices of parallel imported products "are on average the same as those of locally sourced equivalents . . ." (despite average price differentials of more than 20 percent). Parallel trade in Europe involves trade between pharmacies and wholesalers subject to regulations in their respective home markets. It does *not* involve individuals importing medicines on their own from foreign jurisdictions. Our long experience analyzing parallel trade and considerable objective research shows the gains ultimately accrue to the middlemen rather than to consumers or payers.

The issue of importation and how it may impact the safety of American patients is a serious health issue *requiring* informed debate. In 1987, Congress enacted important changes to prohibit the importation of unapproved medicines in response to many instances of unsafe foreign medicines entering the United States. While the public health threats caused by such medications were significant enough in 1987, the potential threats from unapproved prescription drugs are even greater today.

Here are a few key points that we believe need to be factored into the discussion:

• Unapproved, unregulated and counterfeit medicines bought online can (and do) come from virtually anywhere in the world. In light of the counterfeiting activity Pfizer has investigated, the importation proposals we have seen in Washington and some of the States are truly alarming. These programs open a tightly regulated system to a new drug distribution channel in which virtually every participant operates outside the law, outside the standards of acceptable medical practice and without effective oversight.

• In December 2003, the Minnesota Board of Pharmacy investigated eight Canadian Internet pharmacies and found 32 different unsafe or questionable pharmacy practices (on pre-arranged visits!), including unsupervised technicians performing pharmacist functions; shipping multiple labels unattached from multiple prescriptions in the same box; incomplete patient profiles; returned products re-labeled and resold; and unsafe storage and shipping, particularly of temperature-sensitive drugs. The Board investigators found that the standards followed by the Canadian Internet export operations varied greatly from pharmacy to pharmacy—some "appearing to have few standards at all."[1]

• A still larger concern is that consumers don't have any real idea about the true origin of the products. As the National Association of Boards of Pharmacy cautioned in its Position Paper on importation:[2] "An order for what is purported to be a Canadian drug may never be filled by a legitimate Canadian pharmacy with a Canadian drug or even be filled in Canada. The well-known risks that all consumers take when purchasing over the Internet, where, for example, an anonymous company may be 'here today and gone tomorrow' or an illicit business is disguised as a legitimate organization, are heightened when purchasing foreign drugs."

• This concern is echoed in *Prevention* magazine's detailed review of Internet pharmacy practices: "Shoppers need to be aware of a deceptive tactic known as 'hiding under the maple leaf': Web sites that advertise themselves as Canadian or prominently display the familiar maple leaf flag but are actually registered elsewhere."[3]

• The dangerous nature of the products being shipped from foreign Internet pharmacies across the American border is exemplified by recent spot examinations conducted by the FDA and U.S. Customs. These found many shipments containing dangerous, unapproved and counterfeit drugs that pose serious safety problems. An overwhelming majority of the parcels violated U.S. laws and regulations because they contained unapproved drugs."

Finally, a study by the head of the University of Michigan School of Public Health's Department of Health Management and Policy warns that Federal drug importation would result in the loss to the State of thousands of jobs, decreased availability of U.S.-discovered medicines around the world, and diminished patient health benefits as a result of reduced future availability of new medicines from an overall reduction in R&D.[4]

---

[1] Minnesota Board of Pharmacy Office Memorandum, at 2–5 (December 24, 2003).

[2] "National Association of Boards of Pharmacy Position Paper on the Importation of Foreign Prescription Drugs, March 2003.

[3] "No Prescription? No Problem," Prevention.com *http://www.prevention.com/cda/feature2002/0,2479,s1-6568,00.html#top.*

[4] "Prescription Drug Importation, Investment and Employment in Michigan," Dean G. Smith, Ph.D., Professor and Chair of the Department of Health Management and Policy, School of Public Health, University of Michigan, Sept. 21, 2004.

The situation overseas is no better. Notably, in recent months the UK suffered two high-profile counterfeit cases involving fake medicines in the legitimate supply chain:[5]

• In August, a UK health care agency issued an alert recalling two batches of Lilly's Cialis when counterfeits were discovered after a patient reported to Lilly that his 20mg tablets were crumbly.

• In September, the same UK agency issued a second alert recalling a batch of Abbott's Reductil after counterfeits were spotted by a wholesaler after it became suspicious of the batch number.

The extent of counterfeit medicines in the UK is unclear. However, at the end of 2000, the Centre for Economic Business Research claimed that 6 percent of the drugs in the UK were probably fake.[6] Pfizer believes that international counterfeit operations are clearly targeting Europe's legitimate supply system.

We hope you will take this information and the issues they raise into consideration as your committee considers this important issue.

Sincerely,

CHUCK HARDWICK,
Senior Vice President,
Worldwide Government & Public Affairs.

The CHAIRMAN. Thank you all for appearing here today. We will look forward to your further answers.

[**Editors Note—Due to the high cost of printing, previously published materials submitted by witnesses are maintained in the committee files.**]

[Additional material follows.]

---

[5] "Counterfeit Drugs Set Alarm Bells Ringing," Pharmaceutical Journal, 11 September 2004, p1.

[6] "Fake medicines cost £180m, says ACG," Pharmaceutical Journal, 23/30 December 2000, p. 905.

ADDITIONAL MATERIAL

PREPARED STATEMENT OF SENATOR VITTER

Mr. Chairman, I welcome the opportunity to discuss the issue of prescription drug importation. This is an issue about which I feel strongly: my first legislative action as a U.S. Senator was to introduce the Pharmaceutical Market Access Act of 2005 (S. 109).

I would have to say that introducing S. 109, which would put affordable prescription drugs within reach of all Americans, was not an easy first action. This bipartisan bill is opposed by some very powerful interests in Washington, including the big drug companies. The bill is opposed by the Administration and it was not particularly welcomed by any leadership in Congress, Senate or House, Republican or Democrat. But I could not ignore the wishes of a vast majority of the citizens of my State.

As I traveled throughout Louisiana over the past year, I heard countless seniors in particular tell similar stories about the outrageous costs of their prescription drugs and how it burdens their lives. The United States is the world's largest market for pharmaceuticals. Yet we pay the world's highest prices. American seniors alone will spend $1.8 trillion on prescription drugs over the next decade. Meanwhile, citizens of virtually every other industrialized country pay significantly lower prices, lower by 30 percent or more. And this figure includes many countries which are not dominated by old-fashioned price control regimes.

My bill would make prescription drugs more affordable by expanding free trade and world commerce, by legalizing the importation of prescription drugs from 25 industrialized countries with pharmaceutical structures equivalent or superior to our own. For the first time, individual consumers would be allowed to legally import prescription drugs for their personal use.

Critics of drug importation cite safety as their primary concern. I share a belief that the safety of prescription drugs is paramount. My bill takes steps to resolve real safety concerns and strengthen existing laws by adding new requirements to promote the safety of prescription drugs here at home and those brought in from abroad. It includes new requirements that imported prescription drugs either be packaged and shipped using state-of-the-art counterfeit-resistant technologies or be carefully tested for authenticity before entering commerce in our country.

Not long ago, a team of specialists, appointed by the Governor of Illinois, exhaustively researched the question of whether Americans can safely and effectively purchase prescription drugs from other industrialized countries. Their findings are described in two recent reports: the first, entitled "Report on Feasibility of Employees and Retirees Safely and Effectively Purchasing Prescription Drugs From Canadian Pharmacies" (released October 27, 2003); and the second, entitled "Can Illinois Residents and Businesses Safely and Effectively Purchase Prescription Drugs From Europe" (released June 28, 2004).

The authors of the first report conclude that Canadian methods of ensuring the safety and efficacy of prescription drugs are comparable to those of the United States. As noted in the October 27, 2003 report, at virtually every level, the United States and Canada have comparable requirements for the warehousing and storage of pharmaceuticals. The authors also conclude that Canada's system for the pricing and distribution of prescription drugs is less likely to foster drug counterfeiting than our own system in the United States.

The authors of the second report conclude that it is both possible and desirable to allow purchases of prescription drugs from approved facilities in Europe; and they say it can be done in a manner that protects consumer safety. The authors also predict that consumer cost-savings can be achieved if drug companies do not restrict or stop supplies to foreign facilities that sell prescription drugs to Americans. Finally, the report details how residents of the United States spend more money on health care than residents of any other country in the world, yet the higher spending does not guarantee lower mortality rates or longer life expectancies. I request that the full text of both reports be included in the Record of this hearing with my statement.

Drug importation is not a conservative or liberal issue. It is not a Democrat or Republican issue. It is a universal issue and a challenge to provide our Nation's consumers access to safe and affordable drugs. That is why I worked to assemble a coalition of Senators and Representatives from across the political spectrum in support of this legislation. This coalition makes the bill unique as the first bipartisan and bicameral drug importation proposal.

On January 25, 2005, U.S. Congressman Gil Gutknecht introduced the companion measure to S. 109 in the House of Representatives. His bill, H.R. 328, is identical to the one that I introduced on January 24th; and, like my bill, it has bipartisan support. An earlier version of the Gutknecht bill passed the House of Representatives in the 108th Congress with my strong support and it remains the only bill ever to pass either chamber on this subject. Congressman Gutknecht and I share the view that an unaffordable drug is neither safe nor effective.

I look forward to working with all of my new Senate colleagues to advance the cause of drug importation for all Americans. And, of course, my door is always open to those who want to join our effort or who have other ideas on how to bring the high cost of prescription drugs down to an affordable level. This issue is too important for us not to act.

Prepared Statement of the American Pharmacists Association (APhA)

The American Pharmacists Association (APhA) appreciates the opportunity to provide our perspective on the risks and benefits associated with prescription drug importation. APhA, founded in 1852 as the American Pharmaceutical Association, represents more than 52,000 practicing pharmacists, pharmaceutical scientists, student pharmacists, and pharmacy technicians. APhA is the first-established and largest national association of pharmacists in the United States.

THE LIKELY RISKS OF PRESCRIPTION DRUG IMPORTATION

The public pressure to address access to lower prescription prices has prompted Congress to look at the possibility of legalizing prescription drug importation. This charge carries with it a significant responsibility—to determine if prescription drug importation can be conducted safely, and its potential impact on public health, medical costs, and the development of new medications. To make this determination, Congress must consider a number of important questions ranging from the scope and volume of imported drugs, the adequacy of safety protections, and potential liability issues, to the need for modifications in manufacturing and distribution technologies, the drug distribution system, and State and Federal laws.

We appreciate why many have rallied around importation as the "solution" to providing consumers access to lower cost prescription drugs. As pharmacists, we are acutely aware that some patients—especially seniors—face challenges in accessing valuable, but sometimes unaffordable, medications. Many pharmacists can vividly recall the dismay of having to tell one of their patients—especially a senior on a fixed income—the cost of their medication, knowing that the cost may be more than the patient can afford. Consequently, APhA strongly supports efforts to enhance patient access to prescription medications. However, we have significant concerns with proposals to "solve" the problem by expanding importation. Our concerns generally fit in two areas: the integrity of the drug product itself and the impact on patient care.

THE INTEGRITY OF THE MEDICATION

The current U.S. drug distribution system was designed to keep unapproved and potentially unsafe medications from entering the U.S. drug supply. Current U.S. laws and regulations were put in place after several critical incidents resulted in patient harm. When patients were harmed by contaminated or ineffective medications, Congress took action to protect patients. Those actions included requiring evidence of safety and effectiveness, controlling the production and distribution of products, prohibiting the importation of unapproved medications, and other efforts to limit the presence of counterfeit and contaminated medications. Intentionally circumventing the U.S. regulatory system—as prescription drug importation would allow—creates an opportunity for mislabeled, mishandled, subpotent, or counterfeit drugs to make their way onto the shelves of pharmacies and into the hands of patients.

In an attempt to reduce the risk, some Congressional proposals have limited importation to specific countries. While some countries, such as Canada, may have a system to regulate medications comparable to the U.S. system, it is important to recognize that a program limited to import prescription drugs from Canada—no matter how carefully designed—will open the closed U.S. regulatory system to countries beyond Canada. "Opening the door" to Canada opens the door—period. And opening the door creates opportunities for unscrupulous operators to penetrate the system. Before any new system is adopted, we must be certain that, at a minimum, U.S. regulatory authorities will be able to distinguish between a "legitimate" (a prescription filled through an "approved" importation program) package of prescription drugs crossing the U.S. border and another package of prescription drugs entering the United States from an unapproved country or drug seller.

It's also critical to keep in mind that while Canada is touted most frequently as the source of the imported products, there are no guarantees that the drugs U.S. patients will receive are those that are being delivered to Canadian citizens. In fact, as reports have indicated, Canada is not equipped to handle the demand that would potentially occur if prescription drug importation was legalized in America. The Internet pharmacies that are currently filling most of the orders—in violation of U.S. law—are now threatening to move to other countries to increase their supplies of drugs. Without a comprehensive, well-structured, well-funded new bureaucracy to regulate prescription drug importation, American patients, pharmacists, and physicians will have no guarantee that the products that physicians prescribe, pharmacists dispense and work with, and patients ingest won't do more harm to the patient than good.

But even *with* the comprehensive U.S. system, counterfeit drugs have penetrated our system. According to the Food and Drug Administration (FDA), the number of counterfeit drug investigations has increased fourfold since the late 1990's.[1] For example, in 2003, 11,000 boxes of counterfeit Epogen and Procrit were found on pharmacy shelves and in patients' homes. Three months later, the FDA discovered five lots of counterfeit Lipitor. And more recently, the FDA warned of counterfeit Ortho Evra contraceptive patches that contain no active ingredient and were being sold online by a company based in India. These examples support the need for review and refinement of our existing safety net, not the expansion of efforts to circumvent or relax that system. A poorly constructed importation proposal would relax our current system and damage our safety net. Opening the door to importation increases the risk of counterfeit medications infiltrating our drug supply.

Even when a patient receives a "legitimate" drug, there are differences between drugs that are sold in the United States and other countries. Medications obtained outside of the United States may contain different formulations—with differences in the amount of active ingredient or differences in the type of inactive ingredients—both of which can affect the product's stability and how the product works. Because of these differences, any safe importation system must limit importation to products approved by the Food and Drug Administration, not merely products that contain the same, or similar, active ingredients. Medications are different—and minor differences matter.

Storage and shipping conditions can also affect drug stability and potency. Consumers who obtain their medications outside the United States have no way to know how their medications were handled. Any safe importation system must ensure that the medication was maintained at the correct temperature, was stored in the correct type of container, and was properly protected during shipment.

IMPACT ON PATIENT CARE

Importation not only removes the United States guarantee to patients that their drugs will be safe, it also directly impacts patient care. While much of the importation debate is driven by disparities in drug pricing, those disparities are evident only on the front end—when we only know the cost of the drug, not the value. The most expensive medication is the one that doesn't work: in the situation where the drug doesn't lower blood pressure appropriately, the consumer paid good money, but received no benefit. In addition to paying cash, the patient paid a price with their health as their condition went unmanaged. The value of a medication should be assessed after the consumer has used it, after consultation with their pharmacist and doctor to make the best use of it. But this collaboration is challenged in many importation scenarios.

Because of the stigma involved in importing medications, many patients do not tell their physician or pharmacist about medications they are securing outside of the United States. This is understandable, but dangerous. When a patient obtains medications from multiple sources—in this case through importation and a local pharmacy—neither the domestic nor international pharmacist has the patient's complete medication profile unless the patient provides this information. The pharmacist is unable to determine whether the new prescription will conflict with any other medications the patient takes, whether the new prescription has ingredients that duplicate a current prescription, or whether its mere presence suggests other medical problems for the patient that should be followed-up with the patient's physician. This virtual blindness compromises the ability of physicians to care for their patients and the ability of pharmacists to partner with patients to improve medication use and advance patient care.

[1] William Hubbard. Statement before the Senate Committee on Finance Subcommittee on Health Care and Subcommittee on International Trade. April 27, 2004.

Not knowing a patient's entire medication regimen or the content and strength of a particular drug can also cause problems when a patient suffers unexpected complications or does not respond as expected to a medication. Consider a patient working with their local physician and pharmacist to treat their high blood pressure. The patient imports a faulty medication that has no, or little, active ingredient. It is unlikely the patient will physically feel anything different; it is unlikely he would actually notice any difference in the product. Later the patient visits the physician and his blood-pressure reading shows that the medication is not working. Because of our trust in the medication supply, it is highly unlikely that the physician will consider that there was a problem with the medication. Rather, the physician will likely assume that the medication did not work and will consequently either increase the dose or choose another medication. This sets the stage for using a stronger, but potentially unnecessary, medication and increasing overall health care costs.

Also consider the scenario where a patient is in need of a prescription medication on a short timeframe—such as an antibiotic for an infection or a pain medication to treat symptoms from an injury. If that patient has been importing his or her medications, the pharmacist is unable to determine whether the new prescription will conflict with any other medications the patient takes, has ingredients that duplicate a current prescription, or whether its mere presence suggests other medical problems for the patient that should be followed-up with the patient's physicians. This "blindness" compromises the ability of physicians to care for their patients and the ability of pharmacists to partner with patients to improve medication use and advance patient care.

Both of these scenarios help explain why it is difficult to answer the often asked question, "Where are the bodies [the documented evidence of patient harm from importation]?" Counterfeit drugs can exacerbate illness and/or hasten death. But it's unlikely that either of these results would be linked to a faulty drug because of our current faith in the U.S. drug supply. Importation could cloud the promise of improved health from medications; importation compromises the pharmacist's role in patient care.

THE NEED TO ADDRESS ISSUES OF CONCERN

Medications have become a critical aspect of patient care. But prescription medications are only safe and effective when patients receive "what the doctor ordered", understand how to use the drug appropriately, and what side effects they should watch. Direct interaction between the prescribers, pharmacists and patients is critical to ensuring appropriate medication use. Effective patient care is about real relationships—physician-patient, pharmacist-physician, and pharmacist-patient relationships. To remove such a basic component of our health care delivery system's safety net seems diametrically opposed to the "pro patient safety" environment we are all working to achieve.

When you consider all of the risks associated with the importation of prescription drugs, just a few of which have been described, it appears foolhardy to consider haphazardly opening our borders to imported pharmaceuticals. Allowing importation carries the risk that mislabeled, mishandled, subpotent, or counterfeit drugs will reach the hands of U.S. patients. We suggest that Congress stop asking the question "do we allow importation?", which has become highly politicized, and instead ask "what do we do to assure the safety and the integrity of the U.S. drug supply?"

There appear to be two options. One, we begin strictly enforcing current law that prohibits importation. Provide the FDA, the Drug Enforcement Administration, Customs Bureau, and other regulatory agencies the funds and resources necessary to enforce the law; and continue efforts to find other means of increasing access to affordable medications. At a minimum, policymakers should avoid any further endorsement of this unregulated and unknown practice. Instead, we must continue to educate consumers on the risks.

The second option is developing a new bureaucracy to assure the safety of our medication supply. A new system, regardless of whether or not it allows importation, must resolve several issues of concern to ensure that patients continue to receive safe and effective medications—and that they know how to use those medications. Specifically, a new system must address the role of the FDA and the State Boards of Pharmacy in maintaining a safe drug supply, respect the patient-pharmacist-physician relationship, require valid prescriptions, assure consumer recourse for harm, prevent efforts to circumvent U.S. health care professionals, include measures to limit counterfeit and contaminated drugs, and address the differences between FDA-approved medications and foreign products. Even this long litany of issues is not an exhaustive list of what must be tackled when evaluating a system to protect the U.S. drug supply and American consumers.

BALANCING RISK AND BENEFIT

Prescription drugs, unlike so many other products, are not just another commodity—we ingest them to affect our bodies. They are one of the most valuable weapons we have in our health care arsenal today and we must treat them as such. Pharmacists rely on the quality of the U.S. prescription drug supply to provide their patients with safe and effective treatments. As the FDA does when it evaluates a new prescription drug, we must look at both the risks and the benefits and determine if the benefits outweigh the risks.

Importation may provide the benefit of lower cost prescription drugs, but as currently practiced it appears that the benefits do not outweigh the potential risks. We caution against recommending importation as an alternative method of drug distribution without appropriate safeguards—both in statute or regulation and in enforcement. At a minimum, any legalization of importation should be limited to drug products approved by the Food and Drug Administration and assure coordination of care with the consumer's doctor and pharmacist. The perils of personal importation via the Internet are many. If our closed system is opened, we must have strong measures—and enforcement behind those measures—to help decrease the likelihood of unscrupulous operators preying on consumers through their medicine cabinet.

APhA thanks you for the opportunity to provide comments on this important issue. We appreciate the committee's commitment to examining the wide range of issues surrounding the prescription drug importation debate. We offer our assistance to the committee as you continue your valuable work to develop a safe and effective system of providing prescription medications and pharmacists' services to all Americans.

PREPARED STATEMENT OF ALLERGAN, INC.

This testimony is submitted on behalf of Allergan, Inc., a biologics and pharmaceutical company headquartered in Irvine, California. Allergan develops innovative therapies for vision, muscular, and other disorders and conditions. We have developed a number of orphan products, including Botox, which is a biologic used to treat dystonia and related eye disorders, as well as muscular contracture in pediatric cerebral palsy patients.

We appreciate the opportunity to submit testimony on the matter of prescription drug importation legislation, and in particular, on the need for an exemption in such legislation for FDA-designated orphan drugs. Allergan believes that Congress should exclude orphan drugs from prescription drug importation legislation for two reasons: (1) permitting importation of orphan drugs would endanger patient safety, as many orphan drugs have unique handling requirements which are critical for maintaining their potency; and (2) permitting importation of orphan drugs would undermine the Orphan Drug Act and thus jeopardize the future development of rare disease therapies.

I. BACKGROUND ON ORPHAN DRUGS

"Orphan" drugs are drugs (including biologicals) that are developed specifically to treat a rare disease or condition, *i.e.*, generally, a disease or condition that affects fewer than 200,000 people nationwide. According to the National Organization for Rare Disorders, more than 6,000 rare diseases have been identified. Some rare diseases are as familiar as cystic fibrosis, hemophilia, and Lou Gehrig's disease, while others—such as Hamburger disease and Job syndrome—might be known only to the relative few who are afflicted with the disease, along with their families and health care professionals. By definition, the number of people with a particular orphan disease is relatively small, but collectively, rare diseases afflict more than 25 million Americans. In fact, 1 out of every 10 people in the United States has received a rare disease diagnosis. Rare disease patients rely on orphan drugs to treat their diseases, which often are life-threatening acute or chronic conditions.

II. IMPORTATION OF ORPHAN DRUGS WOULD ENDANGER PATIENT SAFETY

Exempting orphan drugs from prescription drug importation legislation is imperative to ensure the safety of rare disease therapies administered in the United States. Many orphan drugs are biologicals, which often require unique handling and shipping measures, such as maintaining the product at specific and sometimes extreme temperatures, and limiting the product's exposure to light. These unique handling requirements are critical to maintaining the product's safety and efficacy. The failure to adhere to these special handling requirements can endanger patient health by making the product ineffective or even harmful. However, it is difficult, if not impossible, to determine whether and the extent to which a drug's potency has been compromised as a result of failure to adhere to prescribed shipping requirements.

The dosage form of many orphan drugs makes them particularly vulnerable to unscrupulous counterfeiters. Many orphan drugs are infused or injected. The liquid form of these infused and injectable products makes them more susceptible to counterfeiting than tablets or pills—and more dangerous for patients. These products are infused and injected directly into the bloodstream, and thus, the effects of counterfeit drugs are experienced immediately and severely.

These safety concerns are not hypothetical or exaggerated. Consider the following reported examples of counterfeit or diluted orphan drugs that have entered the U.S. drug supply under current law:

- *Epogen (epoetin alfa).* Epogen is an injectable biologic used to stimulate red blood cell production. On February 21, 2001, the manufacturer of Epogen disclosed reported incidents of tampering. The flip caps from some vials had been removed and the vial contents were replaced with varying amounts of a subpotent aqueous solution. The vials bore counterfeit labels with phony lot numbers. Lab tests revealed that some vials contained active ingredient 20 times lower than expected. A 16-year-old liver transplant patient suffered severe muscle cramping after receiving injections of the subpotent drug. His parents had purchased the drug from a national pharmacy chain store, which had in turn received it from one of three national drug distributors.
- *Gamimune N (immune globulin intravenous, human).* Gamimune N is a liquid formulation plasma concentrate used to treat various immune deficiencies. In early 2002, nurses noticed that certain vials of Gamimune N were atypically cloudy. The manufacturer of Gamimune N recalled two separate lots of the drug, one on February 1, 2002, and one on March 14, 2002. An analysis revealed that someone had tampered with the overseals of at least 13 vials. The damaged vials contained diluted Gamimune N, were contaminated with bacteria, had an unexpectedly low protein concentration, and demonstrated an elevated chloride level.
- *Neupogen (filgrastim).* Neupogen is an injectable colon-stimulating factor used mostly in cancer patients. In 2001, a distributor discovered counterfeit vials of the drug that contained fake lot numbers and incorrect expiration dates. Laboratory tests later revealed that the vials contained only saline solution.
- *Nutropin AQ (somatropin (rDNA origin) infection).* Nutropin AQ is the liquid formulation of Nutropin, a lyophilized recombinant human growth hormone. Nutropin AQ is used to treat children with growth failure and patients suffering from AIDS wasting. In 2001, patients, doctors, and pharmacists detected abnormal vials of Nutropin AQ. Subsequent analysis revealed at least one vial contained insulin instead of Nutropin.
- *Procrit (epoetin alfa).* Procrit helps anemic cancer and HIV patients increase their red blood cell counts. Counterfeit versions of the drug were first discovered in 2002 and have been found at two large wholesalers and a number of retail outlets. Counterfeit lots of the drug that purported to contain 40,000 units only had 2,000 units. Instead of active ingredients, some vials contained bacteria-tainted water that can cause blood stream infections.
- *Retrovir (zidovudine).* Retrovir, also known as AZT, was the first drug approved for the treatment of HIV. In 2001, a routine inspection revealed 52 bottles of counterfeit Retrovir. A spokesperson for the company that had sold the counterfeit drug apologized, explaining that the large volume of sales prevented the adequate detection of counterfeit drugs.
- *Serostim (somatropin (rDNA origin) for injection).* There have been two counterfeit incidents associated with Serostim for injection, a growth hormone used to treat AIDS wasting. In 2001, a recall at the distributor level was prompted by consumer complaints about adverse events. In 2002, the manufacturer of the drug became aware of another counterfeit batch. One batch reportedly contained a generic hormone, while the other contained a significantly smaller dose of the human growth hormone.

Although prescription drug importation legislation may establish safeguards to protect the Nation's drug supply, *safeguards can never be completely effective.* Even the legal safeguards currently in place have not prevented numerous cases of counterfeit and adulterated orphan drugs in the United States. Importation of orphan drugs would only increase the risk of exposing rare disease patients to an ineffective or harmful drug, because more entities that are far beyond the effective control of FDA will handle the drug before it reaches the patient. This introduces a much greater risk that a drug may be mishandled, contaminated, or counterfeited by an unscrupulous or careless person willing to exploit or ignore patient safety for economic benefit. Congress therefore should exempt orphan drugs—with their higher threat of adulteration and contamination, or compromised safety or efficacy due to mishandling—to reduce the risk of introducing unsafe products into the U.S. drug supply.

III. IMPORTATION OF ORPHAN DRUGS WOULD JEOPARDIZE FUTURE DEVELOPMENT OF RARE DISEASE THERAPIES

In enacting the Orphan Drug Act in 1983, Congress recognized the unique challenges that rare diseases pose for patients and drug manufacturers. Congress determined that there are "many diseases and conditions . . . which affect . . . small numbers of individuals," and that "because so few individuals are affected by any one rare disease or condition," companies that develop "orphan drugs" to treat these diseases may "reasonably expect . . . to incur a financial loss" in doing so. Given the inability of companies to recoup costs incurred in bringing these products to market, Congress found that "orphan drugs will not be developed" absent changes in Federal law to encourage their development.

To address this problem, Congress established certain incentives under Federal law for orphan drug development, including market exclusivity for 7 years, tax credits, assistance for clinical research, and research grants. These incentives have been essential to the development of orphan drugs. As a result of the Orphan Dug Act, more than 240 orphan drugs have been developed to treat rare diseases affecting approximately 12 million Americans.

Permitting importation of orphan drugs would thwart the goals of Orphan Drug Act, because it would introduce competition during the period in which the Orphan Drug Act promises market exclusivity. In addition to breaching the promise that Congress made in the Orphan Drug Act, this would impair manufacturers' ability to recover the costs incurred in developing rare disease therapies and discourage future research and development efforts aimed at discovering treatments for rare diseases. This result is precisely what the Orphan Drug Act sought to avoid, and could have disastrous consequences for the future development of orphan drugs—and thus for the millions of Americans suffering from rare diseases for which effective treatments have not yet been developed.

IV. CONCLUSION

In conclusion, we believe it is imperative that Congress exempt orphan drugs from prescription drug importation legislation to ensure the safety of rare disease therapies administered in the United States, and to maintain appropriate incentives to encourage the future development of orphan drugs. Allergan has long been a supporter of the rare disease community and the Orphan Drug Program, and we remain committed to developing innovative therapies for the 25 million Americans suffering from rare diseases. We would be happy to provide the committee with any additional information that may be useful as it considers these important issues.

RESPONSE TO QUESTIONS OF SENATOR KENNEDY BY RICHARD CARMONA, M.D.

Question 1. The HHS Report explains that drug importation would reduce revenues for the drug industry, which would cause them to cut research and development, leading to fewer drugs on the market in the future, and huge societal costs. Instead, the report suggests we find ways to encourage people to use generics whenever available, saying that would save as much or more anyway. Wouldn't switching to generics also decrease revenues for the drug industry, and have the same negative effect on R&D?

Answer 1. While both drug importation and switching to generics would reduce revenue to innovator drug companies, the impacts on future research and development (R&D) are quite different. Many of the drugs likely to be imported are early in their life cycle and are just beginning to repay innovators for their substantial investments. Reductions in revenues in these cases are important because they occur relatively soon after decisions to undertake research and development. When a consumer switches to a generic version of an innovator's drug, however, the reduction in revenues occur later in the life of the innovator's drug—after the expiration of all patents and exclusive marketing opportunities granted by the government. These reductions in revenues are so long after R&D decisions that they are relatively unimportant from the perspective of potential investors in R&D. Thus, we believe the impacts on R&D from increased generic utilization would be minimal. By encouraging consumers to switch to generics whenever available, we are encouraging them to save money while still providing firms bringing costly innovations to market a fair opportunity to recoup their investments.

Question 2. In your testimony you stated that America would likely save less than 1 percent of our total drug bill through importation. That is based in large part on the fact that much of our expenditures are for drugs that are biologics, or generics, or drugs otherwise inappropriate for importation. But, page 75 of the report seems to state that for drugs that would be eligible for importation, "discounts to U.S. drug purchasers will average 20 percent of the price of equivalent U.S. pharmaceutical products." Do you agree that that would be a substantial savings for many individuals, similar to what seniors are receiving with Medicare drug discount cards?

Answer 2. The estimate of 20 percent savings would apply to those drugs eligible for importation, where there would exist an importable supply, and to the extent that intermediaries would not capture more than half of the potential savings. But note that the report states that the discounts would accrue to U.S. "drug purchasers." This is an important distinction. There is no guarantee that individual consumers, in particular cash-paying seniors, would have direct access to these cheaper drugs. The Task Force Report recognizes that, given the economic power of large purchasers, it is possible that all of the available supply could be purchased by large organizations or third-party payers and that few savings would ever reach the individual consumer. While CMS can speak better about the details of the Medicare drug discount cards, it would seem that this program puts the buying power of large groups into the hands of individual consumers, who would have access to cheaper drugs without regard to importable supply or the market power of intermediaries. So one would expect the savings for individual consumers from legalized commercial importation to be quite different from the Medicare drug benefits.

RESPONSE TO QUESTIONS OF SENATOR HATCH BY RICHARD CARMONA, M.D.

Question 1. You mentioned that there are significant safety concerns regarding drug importation, but if Congress wants to legislate a system, it should be closed, well-defined, and capable of ensuring the pedigree of the drugs. While these seem to be valid principles if there were to be an import regime, I am concerned about the practicality of designing a system to meet those requirements. Could you elaborate on what you meant by a closed system? For example, would other countries have to participate? If so, how would the United States negotiate the agreement with those other countries? How would this be enforced? Similarly, what are the ways in which the United States would go about ensuring that pedigree?

Answer 1. The drug distribution network for legal prescription drugs in the United States is a "closed" system that involves several entities (e.g., manufacturers, wholesalers, pharmacies) that move drug products from the point of manufacture to the end user, and provides against receiving unsafe, ineffective, or poor quality medications. All of these entities are known and subject to Federal and State regulatory and legislative oversight. This system evolved as a result of legislative requirements that drugs be treated as potentially dangerous consumer goods that require professional oversight to protect the public health. The result has been a level of safety for drug products that is widely recognized as the world's "gold standard." To maintain current levels of safety, the standards that currently exist in the United States (or some equivalent) would need to apply to all foreign drug suppliers who were authorized to sell drugs into the United States under a legalized commercial importation program. Legalized importation of drugs in such a way that creates an opening in the "closed" system will likely result in some increase in risk, as the evidence shows that weaknesses in the oversight of drug regulation and the distribution system have been exploited.

As stated in the Drug Importation Task Force Report, Memoranda of Understanding (MOU) may be needed with the affected countries to ensure effective enforcement of the terms of a new importation system.

Because electronic track and trace technology and capability is still in its infancy, it would be logistically difficult and resource intensive to validate and authenticate paper pedigrees that include, or originate in, a foreign country.

Question 2. The enforcement mechanism is also of great interest to me, especially in reference to Internet pharmacies. Could you please advise the committee as to how the Internet marketplace could be policed so that American consumers could be assured about the safety, efficacy and pedigree of the medications they are receiving? In the United States, for example, pharmaceutical manufacturing plants are registered and regularly inspected, pharmacies are licensed, etc. Would those same regulatory safeguards exist with respect to products distributed through Internet pharmacies?

Answer 2. The Drug Importation Task Force Report noted that there are an increasing number of foreign Internet pharmacies capitalizing on the vulnerability of patients in search of less expensive prescription drugs. The Internet has created a marketplace for the sale of unapproved drugs, prescription drugs dispensed without a valid prescription, drugs of unknown origin, counterfeit drugs, and otherwise substandard drugs. Although there are a number of legitimate and reputable Internet pharmacies in the United States that serve American consumers, there are a considerable number of Internet pharmacies that are not legitimate and that unlawfully sell prescription drugs to American consumers. Unfortunately, it is very easy to set up a webpage that misrepresents the pharmacy's location, the source and country of origin of its drugs, the regulatory status of the drugs (e.g., whether or not FDA-approved), and its compliance with applicable laws and regulations. It is extremely difficult for highly trained investigators to tell the difference between legitimate and illegal sites; it will be even more difficult for consumers to differentiate. Because of the ease with which such Web sites can be established and because the Internet helps obscure their physical location, it would be nearly impossible to monitor, find, or inspect all of these pharmacies.

Furthermore, the volume of packages entering the United States today has been increasing at a steady rate. Under a personal importation program, it would be very difficult to distinguish which of these millions of packages are from "permitted" Internet pharmacies and which are from rogue Web sites, increasing the potential safety risks associated with imported drugs.

There are efforts to help patients identify if an online pharmacy site is appropriately licensed, such as the Verified Internet Pharmacy Practice Site (VIPPS) certification program, run by the National Association of Boards of Pharmacy. Online pharmacies with the VIPPS logo also have successfully completed a rigorous inspection and review.

RESPONSE TO QUESTIONS OF SENATOR ENZI BY CARMEN CATIZONE

Question 1. I am interested in the VIPPS program to certify Internet Pharmacies. Third-party certification has been remarkably successful in other areas. I do note, however, that you have an extensive disclaimer about the information in the VIPPS database, which states that this information is advisory only, and voluntarily supplied by Boards of Pharmacy and the pharmacy site themselves. What level of resources would it take to verify—on an ongoing basis—the information necessary for safe importation of prescription drugs from online pharmacies?

Answer 1. NABP considers the information provided by the VIPPS program as reliable and valid and certifies all such information with the primary source, State licensing authorities. The disclaimers are legal formalities to recognize the legal authority of the State Agencies and to minimize NABP's liability. Our disclaimers are not meant to diminish the validity of the information. The VIPPS program as presently organized verifies information in a manner and to the extent that would be needed for domestic-based pharmacy practice. The verification of foreign-based pharmacy operations would require extensive resources that NABP could not even estimate at this point.

Question 2. The VIPPS program is completely voluntary. How many Internet pharmacies are participating in VIPPS? What fraction of Internet pharmacies does that constitute?

Answer 2. Since its inception approximately 24 sites have received the VIPPS seal. Over time some of the sites have consolidated or ceased operations or lost their VIPPS accreditation. The 24 VIPPS seals awarded represent some 10–12,000 pharmacies in the United States out of approximately 78,000 total pharmacies in the United States. The total number of legitimate pharmacy Web sites is estimated at approximately 150. A number of these Web sites are local pharmacies that do not serve patients outside of their local patient base and utilize the Internet simply to facilitate refill authorizations or provide medication information.

RESPONSE TO QUESTION OF SENATOR ENZI BY JOHN GRAY

HEALTHCARE DISTRIBUTION MANAGEMENT ASSOCIATION (HDMA),
RESTON, VA 20190–5348,
March 15, 2005.

Below is the response of HDMA President and CEO John Gray to the question for the record posed by Chairman Enzi as a follow-up to John's presentation at the committee's February 16th hearing, "Drug Importation: The Realities of Safety and Security." As always, please do not hesitate to contact me if you have any questions.

Question. I have heard a lot about Radio Frequency Identification (RFID). Can you tell me a little more about this technology, and what sort of role it might play in ensuring the pharmaceutical supply chain, both as it stands now and as things might look if the United States were to legalize drug importation?

Answer. The Healthcare Distribution Management (HDMA) strongly believes that technology can serve an important role in securing the Nation's prescription drug supply; however, no single technology can absolutely prevent counterfeiting. Rather, a layering of various strategies can create a significant barrier to entry. We believe technologies employing radio frequency identification (RFID) utilizing electronic product codes (EPC) hold the most promise for tracking, tracing and authenticating a product's movement across the supply chain.

The EPC is a unique number that identifies a specific item in the supply chain. The EPC may also include identifying information such as the manufacturer, product information and a unique serial number. A RFID tag, which is a silicon microchip, smaller than a grain of sand, and an antenna is applied to the items and contains the EPC number. Using RFID technology, the chip "communicates" its number to a "reader" that picks up the signal and records the information. This technology will allow supply chain stakeholders to track the chain of custody (or pedigree) of every unit of medication on an individual basis. By tying each discrete product unit to a unique electronic ID, a product can be tracked electronically through the supply chain.

Furthermore, EPC/RFID technology represents an opportunity to significantly improve efficiencies in managing supplies and inventory. According to a recent HDMA Healthcare Foundation Report entitled, "Adopting EPC in Healthcare: Costs and Benefits," patient safety can be enhanced and efficiencies to the healthcare supply chain can be achieved via the industry-wide adoption of EPC/RFID. EPC/RFID is more efficient and cost-effective than paper pedigrees or alternative electronic tracking methods that do not involve the serialization of individual products. Paper pedigrees have been forged in previous domestic counterfeiting situations. Moreover, paper pedigrees would literally halt the efficient distribution of drugs given the volume of products delivered and the sophisticated automation technology utilized to do so safely and efficiently.

Tremendous progress is being made in the development and adoption of EPC/RFID technology with respect to pharmaceutical products. This is a monumental endeavor that will require close collaboration among all constituents of the healthcare supply chain and will take several years to proliferate the market in the United States. Industry, commercial vendors and government agencies are working together to develop the necessary standards for communication of tagged items across the supply chain. HDMA is working closely with standards development organizations such as EPCglobal to further the awareness, adoption and implementation of EPC in healthcare distribution. While progress is extremely positive, there are many hurdles to overcome including business and technology challenges such as data management issues, interoperability of tags and readers and standards development. HDMA's focus has been to advocate for the adoption of this technology in the United States.

Although the industry is moving forward in the development and adoption of EPC/RFID technology, it will take time and an unwavering commitment on the part of government and each partner in the supply chain to realize adoption of RFID technology in a measured, meaningful and universal way. HDMA members look forward to the support of the committee in ensuring that our laws and regulations continue to support the industry's role in driving adoption of this important and patient safety enhancing technology.

RESPONSE TO QUESTIONS OF SENATOR ENZI BY GOVERNOR TIM PAWLENTY

OFFICE OF GOVERNOR TIM PAWLENTY,
SAINT PAUL, MN 55155,
March 17, 2005.

Hon. MIKE ENZI, *Chairman,*
Committee on Health, Education, Labor, and Pensions,
U.S. Senate,
Washington, DC 20510–6300.

DEAR SENATOR ENZI: Thank you for the opportunity to testify before the U.S. Senate Committee on Health, Education, Labor, and Pensions on February 16th. It was my pleasure to share with you Minnesota's success in supplying Minnesotans with information and assistance in attaining affordable and safe prescription medicines. You and Senator Hatch both requested additional information and analysis about Minnesota RxConnect and Minnesota Advantage Meds. Below are answers to your inquiries.

Question 1. I was intrigued by your description of the RxConnect program. What does the program cost and how is it funded? Does the cost scale with the number of users? In other words, how much would it cost to double the program? Triple it?

Answer 1. The program cost is minimal and is funded from general State revenues. The work done for the MinnesotaRxConnect program was completed by employees of the Minnesota Department of Human Services. Consequently, no additional funds were expended to hire vendors or contractors. The cost of sending State personnel to inspect pharmacies was approximately $10,000. The cost of printing brochures was $2,893.80.

The hard costs for setting up the program for State employees and their dependents, Advantage-meds.com, was also minimal. Several staff members were involved in implementation and an actuary was paid a small amount to provide drug data. All salaries and other costs were paid out of the employee insurance fund. E-mail was used to announce the program to employees, so the communications costs were minimal.

With both programs, the cost does not scale with the number of users. Expanding the program would not significantly increase costs.

Question 2. Recently, many Canadian Internet pharmacies have announced that they are going beyond Canada to get their medicines for American consumers, into countries such as Israel, parts of the EU, New Zealand, etc. In a poll that was released this past fall on importation, support for importation beyond Canada was around 30–40 percent. Do the Internet pharmacies that Minnesota RxConnect has a relationship with in Canada get their medicines from countries other than Canada and if so, is that information disclosed to consumers buying those medicines?

Answer 2. There are really two parts to the answer. Many of the medications used in Canada are imported into Canada from other countries. However, the same thing is true for the United States. Many brand and generic medications are imported into the United States from Europe, Japan, Israel, India and other countries. Those drugs are approved by the FDA and are purchased by U.S. wholesalers, sold to U.S. pharmacies and dispensed by U.S. pharmacists directly to Americans every day. For example, most of the Lipitor dispensed in both Canadian and American pharmacies is made in a manufacturing plant in Ireland.

Similarly, drugs are imported into Canada with the approval of Health Canada and are ultimately dispensed to Canadian citizens. The Canadian Internet pharmacies, of course, dispense those Canadian-approved drugs to U.S. citizens.

Many of the largest pharmaceutical manufacturers are trying to drive Canadian mail-order pharmacies out of business. They are refusing to sell prescription drugs directly to the pharmacies and are threatening to withhold product from wholesalers that do business with the pharmacies. Consequently, some Canadian mail order pharmacies have established relationships with pharmacies in other countries such as the United Kingdom, Australia, New Zealand, Israel and Chile.

Two of the pharmacies affiliated with our Web site have such relationships. Those pharmacies will not send a prescription to be filled by a pharmacy in another country without informing (and getting written permission from) the customer. The Canadian pharmacy still receives the written prescription, verifies that it is valid and appropriate, checks for problems and enters the data into the pharmacy computer system. Using a secure connection, the data is transmitted to the pharmacy in, say, the United Kingdom, where it is checked again by the U.K. pharmacist and physician. The U.K. pharmacy then sends the filled prescription directly to the customer in the United States. Billing is handled by the Canadian pharmacy. In this example, the drug shipped to the U.S. customer would be approved for use in the United Kingdom. Note that the Canadian pharmacy is not buying and importing the drug from the U.K. and then dispensing it to the U.S. citizen. That would be illegal under Canadian law.

Question 3. While you have advocated for allowing Minnesotans to import drugs from pharmacies in Canada, most importation proposals pending at the Federal level allow pharmacists and wholesalers to import drugs from 20 to 25 countries around the world. What is your position on legislation that goes beyond just Canada and goes beyond personal importation?

Answer 3. Employees of the Minnesota Department of Human Services have studied the pharmaceutical distribution system of the United Kingdom. As part of that study, they reviewed the U.K. parallel importation process and were favorably impressed. A large number of drugs used in the U.K. contain the same active ingredient in the same strength as the drugs used in the United States. They are made by the same manufacturer, look the same, have the same brand name and are sometimes made in the same plant—no matter where they are shipped around the world.

A parallel importer in the United Kingdom must be registered by the appropriate regulatory agency. In addition, it must obtain a license for each and every product it wants to import from another European nation. The imported drug must be approved for use in the United Kingdom, in the country from which it is imported and/or by the European Medicines Agency. The parallel importer must keep meticulous records that detail the sales history of each box of drug that is imported—from manufacturer to foreign wholesaler to parallel importer. Products that are imported into the U.K. typically come from Greece, Italy or Spain. Approximately 20 percent of the drugs dispensed to patients in the United Kingdom are parallel imports. Britons don't appear to be suffering adverse consequences due to drugs imported from Greece, Italy and Spain.

European standards for drug manufacturing and distribution appear to be comparable to those used in the United States and certainly rigorous enough to adequately protect patients in Europe. If parallel importation can work so successfully in Europe, there would seem to be no reason to believe that it couldn't work for the United States.

RESPONSE TO QUESTIONS OF SENATOR HATCH BY GOVERNOR PAWLENTY

I understand that Canadian pharmacies on the Internet require customers to sign a waiver absolving the pharmacies of any liability. These waiver forms routinely make U.S. customers waive many other rights, such as the right to privacy, the right to consult a qualified pharmacist, the right to child-proof packaging, and any warranties that the drugs are safe and effective.

Many of these requirements are well-established tenets of U.S. practice and law. For example, the right to privacy of medical information was established by HIPAA, an act passed overwhelmingly by the Congress. The U.S. standard of safety and efficacy for pharmaceuticals is the hallmark of our country's drug approval system, and a requirement that has led many to call our system the "gold standard" of the world.

Question 1. My questions are this: Why should Minnesota consumers be required to waive these important requirements, requirements that largely apply to the purchase of pharmaceuticals in other States? Have you developed any information, such as public education or surveys, to gauge the measure to which your residents are aware of these important rights and the fact that they are entering into legal agreements to waive them, agreements that would in effect make the consumers responsible for the potentially hazardous results of safety problems?

Answer 1. We agree that Minnesota consumers should not be required to sign waivers of liability. The pharmacies affiliated with the MinnesotaRxConnect and Minnesota Advantage-meds Web sites do not require patients to sign waivers of liability.

Question 2. You stated in your testimony that since the launch of MinnesotaRxConnect, not a single complaint has been raised regarding the quality, effectiveness, or safety of the drugs that were purchased utilizing your prescription drug Web site. My questions are this: On what do you base these figures? Would you please describe the post-marketing surveillance system you have put into place?

Answer 2. State agencies have received a number of letters, e-mails and phone calls about the importation programs. No more than 20 have been complaints—with three-fourths of the complaints involving FDA seizure of medications. The remaining complaints were about pricing issues or delayed shipments. We have received no complaints about the quality, effectiveness or safety of drug products.

The pharmacies affiliated with our programs keep internal logs of complaints and we have reviewed them. The complaints most commonly involve billing errors or delayed shipment. In many cases delayed shipments were traced to FDA drug seizures. In a few instances, the wrong drug had been shipped. However, U.S. pharmacies (both mail order and community) sometimes dispense an incorrect medication. Again, we noted no complaints involving the quality, effectiveness or safety of the drug products shipped.

The actions taken by the pharmacies affiliated with our Web sites in response to drug recalls provides further assurance that they take the safety of patients seriously. When Vioxx was voluntarily recalled by the manufacturer, the pharmacies contacted all of the patients to whom they had recently shipped Vioxx to notify them of the recall. They even accepted returns of unused Vioxx. That was at a financial loss because Merck won't accept returns from the Canadian Internet pharmacies.

We have not surveyed users of the MinnesotaRxConnect or Advantage-meds.com Web sites because we do not track them. We feel it would be inappropriate for the State of Minnesota to track the identities and drug usage of the people who use our Web sites.

Thank you again for the opportunity to testify before you. Please do not hesitate to contact me or my staff if you have additional questions about Minnesota programs.

Sincerely,

TIM PAWLENTY,
Governor.

RESPONSE TO QUESTIONS OF THE COMMITTEE BY PETER ROST, M.D.

Question 1. Dr. Rost, you wrote in a January 2005 commentary published in the Star-Ledger that Americans would save $37.8 billion annually from legalized importation. Your findings contradict modeling done by the HHS Task Force, as well as calculations by the Congressional Budget Office, both of whom found savings of about 1–2 percent of total drug spending. As you state in the editorial, your calculations were based on the assumption that legislation to permit importation would also make it illegal to limit supply. What basis do you have to believe that the Congress would support those provisions and that they would pass Constitutional muster?

Answer 1. The house already passed the Pharmaceutical Market Access Act once, (the "Gutknecht bill"), which allow for drug importation to begin without first requiring certification by the Health and Human Services Secretary.

The new, bipartisan Pharmaceutical Market Access and Drug Safety Act introduced by Senator Byron L. Dorgan and others in February 2005 includes a number of provisions intended to ensure that the drug industry cannot thwart the law and prevent consumers from reaping the benefits of drug importation:

- Allows drug importation to begin without first requiring certification by the HHS Secretary.
- Includes a non-discrimination provision that would make it an unfair and discriminatory act for drug manufacturers to get around the law by shutting down the supply of prescription drugs they make available to pharmacists and wholesalers, as they are currently doing in Canada. However, these provisions do not "force" drug companies to sell an unlimited quantity of their products in any given country, nor would drug companies be selling their products for a loss in those countries where they do choose to continue selling their products. Therefore, there is no unconstitutional "takings."
- Also includes features to prevent a drug company from blocking importation by making subtle changes to a drug, such as changing the color or the place of manufacture, so that it is no longer FDA approved.

The Senate bill already has more than 30 cosponsors. Senator Frist blocked the vote of a similar bill in 2004, because he feared it would be approved.

This may be the strongest indication that the bill would pass.

Question 2. What are your calculated savings if these forced sales provisions are NOT included in legislation?

Answer 2. The Congressional Budget Office, when calculating savings of 1–2 percent assumed that pharmaceutical companies would limit supply. The HHS report also states "The foreign supply of patented brand-name drugs may be limited relative to the total volume of such drugs consumed in the U.S. market. Imported drugs may be around 12 percent of total use of such drugs in the United States, depending on the scope of any importation program, because drug companies have incentives to impede exports." This is one key factor resulting in low savings in the HHS report. I agree with the Congressional Budget Office and HHS report that if provisions to guarantee free supply are NOT included in a bill, savings would amount to 1–2 percent of total drug bill, although I believe the HHS report has come to that conclusion using incorrect assumptions.

Average drug prices are 50 percent lower in Europe than in the United States (HHS report, figure 7.2). HHS also assumes that manufacturers will restrict supply, and that "imported drugs may be around 12 percent of total use of such drugs in the United States" I think the number 12 percent is far too high in a scenario in which manufacturers limit supply. More realistic may be around 4–6 percent. The

HHS report also makes the fundamental mistake of assuming that "U.S. drug buyers may get discounts of only 20 percent or less, with the rest of the difference between U.S. and foreign prices going to commercial importers." In my experience, in Europe, parallel trade starts with price differences as low as 8–10 percent and I think it is more realistic to assume that U.S. drug buyers will get discounts of about 40–45 percent. 40 percent discount on 4 percent of total use would result in savings of 1.6 percent annually.

Please also note that the CBO and HHS numbers do not quantify indirect savings that might accrue as a result of drug companies limiting price increases or lowering their U.S. prices domestically in order to make importation less necessary.

Question 3. As you know, the Canadian market is very small relative to the U.S. market. If importation became a widespread practice, how do you envision the Canadian government responding if shortages in their market develop? Do you foresee any problems for Canadian or U.S. patients if that were to occur? Have you considered that even if Congress passes legislation to legalize importation, countries may act to prohibit the export of medicines from their own countries?

Answer 3. Canada alone is not a large enough market and therefore any real drug importation bill does need to allow parallel trade not just with Canada but with other major industrialized nations, particularly the EU. If Congress passes a law that makes limitation of supply illegal, with appropriate penalties, shortages would be avoided. The example to use is Europe, in which the Rome treaty guarantees free trade. Individual countries have laws or trade agreements that ensure that the local market is fully supplied and that only excess drugs are exported. This has created an effective distribution system without supply problems for over 20 years.

Clearly, if drug companies have the opportunity to limit supply, they will. In any such instance local governments are likely to ensure that local supply is not jeopardized. Restricting supply within Europe is illegal, while clearly an increased demand can result in supply restrictions until manufacturing can be increased, which may take 12–24 months. Drug companies already today use this excuse to try to limit supply within EU. A strong U.S. law with appropriate financial penalties could actually alleviate this situation, since it would make it even more difficult for companies to limit production or take a chance on being sued by the European Union.

Question 4. You indicate in your testimony that many Americans cannot afford prescription drugs, and you suggest importation as a solution. However, generics are usually less expensive than brand drugs. In addition, the new Medicare prescription drug benefit will come into full effect shortly, benefiting millions of seniors. There are also a number of national and State programs to provide assistance with drug costs to low-income Americans. Why should Americans look to Europe for imported drugs, when there are often less expensive options here at home?

Answer 4. Generics are an excellent solution, when available. In reality that is only an option for older drugs. It is reasonable for a wealthy country, such as the United States, to provide a system in which all citizens have access to most recent medical advances. The Medicare drug benefit will provide $1,000 for someone with a $4,000 drug bill. That person is still better off importing drugs. Reality is that national and State programs don't work, otherwise the Kaiser Family Foundation couldn't have reported in a 2001 study that 15 percent of uninsured children and 28 percent of uninsured adults had gone without prescription medication because of cost. The journal Diabetes Care reported in February, 2004 on a study of older adults with diabetes. Twenty-eight percent said they went without food or other necessities to pay for drugs. Legalized and regulated reimportation would provide cheaper drugs right at the pharmacy, without forcing patients to make phone calls, write lengthy applications to drug companies, or go on the Internet in search of rebates or less costly drugs.

[Whereupon, at 11:34 a.m., the committee adjourned.]

○